Eating Right & Additional Supplements for Fitness

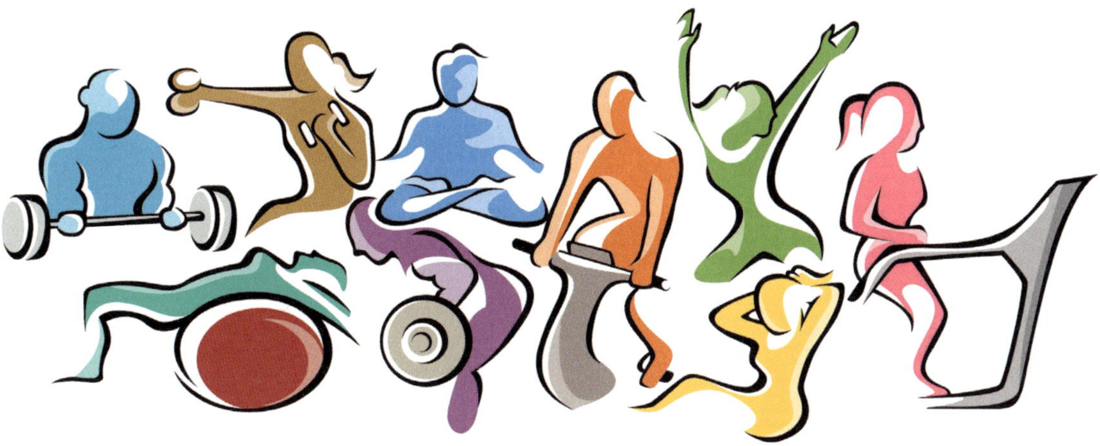

An Integrated Life of Fitness

Core Workouts

Cross-Training

Eating Right & Additional Supplements for Fitness

Endurance & Cardio Training

Exercise for Physical & Mental Health

Flexibility & Agility

Sports & Fitness

Step Aerobics & Aerobic Dance

Weightlifting & Strength Building

Yoga & Pilates

An Integrated
Life of Fitness

Eating Right & Additional Supplements for Fitness

Z.B. HILL

Mason Crest

Mason Crest
450 Parkway Drive, Suite D
Broomall, PA 19008
www.masoncrest.com

Printed and bound in the United States of America.

First printing
9 8 7 6 5 4 3 2 1

Series ISBN: 978-1-4222-3156-2
Hardcover ISBN: 978-1-4222-3159-3
Paperback ISBN: 978-1-4222-3197-5
ebook ISBN: 978-1-4222-8697-5

Cataloging-in-Publication Data on file with the Library of Congress.

CONTENTS

KEY ICONS TO LOOK FOR:

Text-Dependent Questions: These questions send the reader back to the text for more careful attention to the evidence presented there.

Words to Understand: These words with their easy-to-understand definitions will increase the reader's understanding of the text, while building vocabulary skills.

Series Glossary of Key Terms: This back-of-the book glossary contains terminology used throughout this series. Words found here increase the reader's ability to read and comprehend higher-level books and articles in this field.

Research Projects: Readers are pointed toward areas of further inquiry connected to each chapter. Suggestions are provided for projects that encourage deeper research and analysis.

Sidebars: This boxed material within the main text allows readers to build knowledge, gain insights, explore possibilities, and broaden their perspectives by weaving together additional information to provide realistic and holistic perspectives.

INTRODUCTION

Choosing fitness as a priority in your life is one of the smartest decisions you can make! This series of books will give you the tools you need to understand how your decisions about eating, sleeping, and physical activity can affect your health now and in the future.

And speaking of the future: YOU are the future of our world. We who are older are depending on you to build something wonderful—and we, as lifelong advocates of good nutrition and physical activity, want the best for you throughout your whole life.

Our hope in these books is to support and guide you to instill healthy behaviors beginning today. You are in a unique position to adopt healthy habits that will guide you toward better health right now and avoid health-related problems as an adult.

You have the power of choice today. We recognize that it's a very busy world filled with overwhelming choices that sometimes get in the way of you making wise decisions when choosing food or in being active. But no previous training or skills are needed to put this material into practice right away.

We want you to have fun and build your confidence as you read these books. Your self-esteem will increase. LEARN, EXPLORE, and DISCOVER, using the books as your very own personal guide. A tremendous amount of research over the past thirty years has proven that the quality of your health and life will depend on the decisions you make today that affect your body, mind, and inner self.

You are an individual, liking different foods, doing different things, having different interests, and growing up in different families. But you are not alone as you face these vital decisions in your life. Those of us in the fitness professions are working hard to get healthier foods into your schools; to make sure you have an opportunity to be physically active on a regular basis; to ensure that walking and biking are encouraged in your communities; and to build communities where healthy, affordable foods can be purchased close to home. We're doing all we can to support you. We've got your back!

Moving step by step to healthier eating habits and increasing physical activity requires change. Change happens in small steps, so be patient with yourself. Change takes time. But get started *now.*

Lead an "action-packed" life! Your whole body will thank you by becoming stronger and healthier. You can look and do your best. You'll feel good. You'll have more energy. You'll reap the benefits of smart lifestyle choices for a healthier future so you can achieve what's important to you.

Choose to become the best you can be!

—Diana H. Hart, President
National Association for Health and Fitness

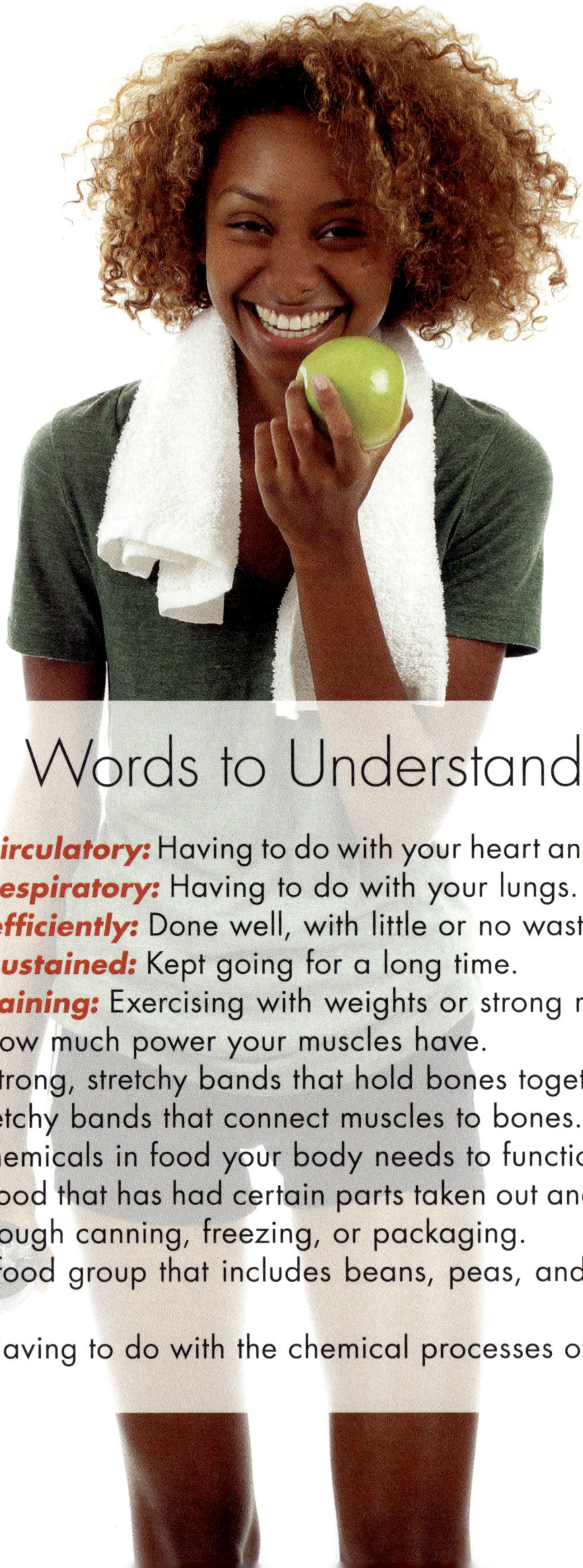

Words to Understand

circulatory: Having to do with your heart and blood vessels.
respiratory: Having to do with your lungs.
efficiently: Done well, with little or no wasted energy.
sustained: Kept going for a long time.
resistance training: Exercising with weights or strong rubber bands to increase how much power your muscles have.
ligaments: Strong, stretchy bands that hold bones together.
tendons: Stretchy bands that connect muscles to bones.
nutrients: Chemicals in food your body needs to function correctly.
processed: Food that has had certain parts taken out and others added, usually through canning, freezing, or packaging.
legumes: A food group that includes beans, peas, and other seeds or pods.
metabolic: Having to do with the chemical processes of your body.

Chapter One

How Are Food and Fitness Connected?

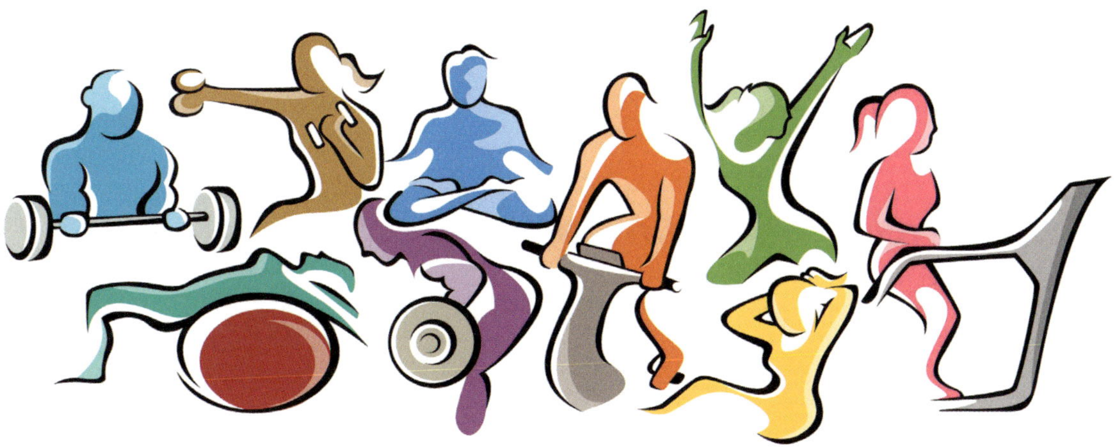

We all have things we want to do. There are places we want to go. Things we want to accomplish. But will we be able to do those things and go those places?

When you are a teen, everything seems possible. It can be hard to think of having physical problems that can prevent you from doing what you want when you want. But if you have diabetes, high blood pressure, or movement issues due to obesity, things you once dreamed about doing may not be possible.

It may not be possible to prevent everything that could get in your way. Illnesses and accidents just happen sometimes. But there are some threats to fitness that can be prevented. And you can start now, while you are still young. Food choices can play a significant role in fitness now and in the future.

WHAT DOES IT MEAN TO BE FIT?

You might think you can tell if someone is fit just by looking at her. But there is more to being physically fit than just looking good.

According to the US Department of Health and Human Services (USDHHS), if someone is physically fit, she has the ability to perform activities. In other words, she can respond well to physically demanding situations, function well in emergencies, be in excellent health, and be able to resist disease and injury. Many experts say that physical fitness is made up of five things.

Cardiorespiratory Endurance

Cardiorespiratory endurance is how our body uses its ***circulatory*** and ***respiratory*** systems to provide fuel during physical activity. Endurance is based on how ***efficiently*** the heart and lungs deliver oxygen throughout the body and how much energy is needed to for muscles to move your bones. The better your lungs and heart send oxygen throughout the body and the less energy needed to for the muscles' movement, the better your fitness.

To increase cardiorespiratory endurance, you should do things that safely cause an increase in heart rate for a ***sustained*** time. Swimming, brisk walking, jogging, playing tennis, and cycling are among the activities that will help increase cardiorespiratory endurance. And you can have fun doing them!

Muscular Strength

According to the USDHHS, muscular strength refers to the muscles' ability to exert force during an activity. ***Resistance training*** is a good

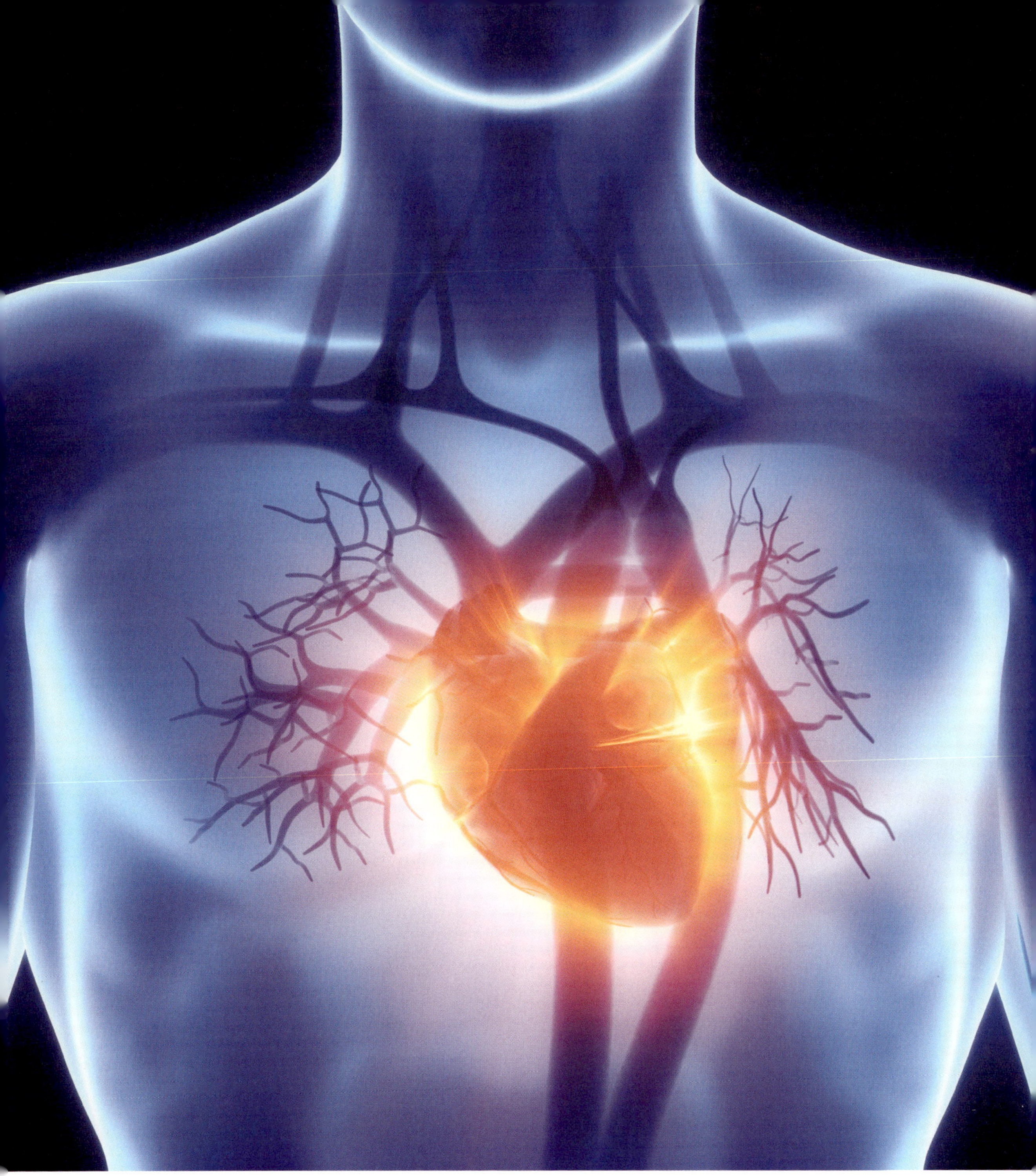

The better your heart works, the more oxygen it can pump to your muscles through your blood. This means your muscles can keep working longer without getting tired.

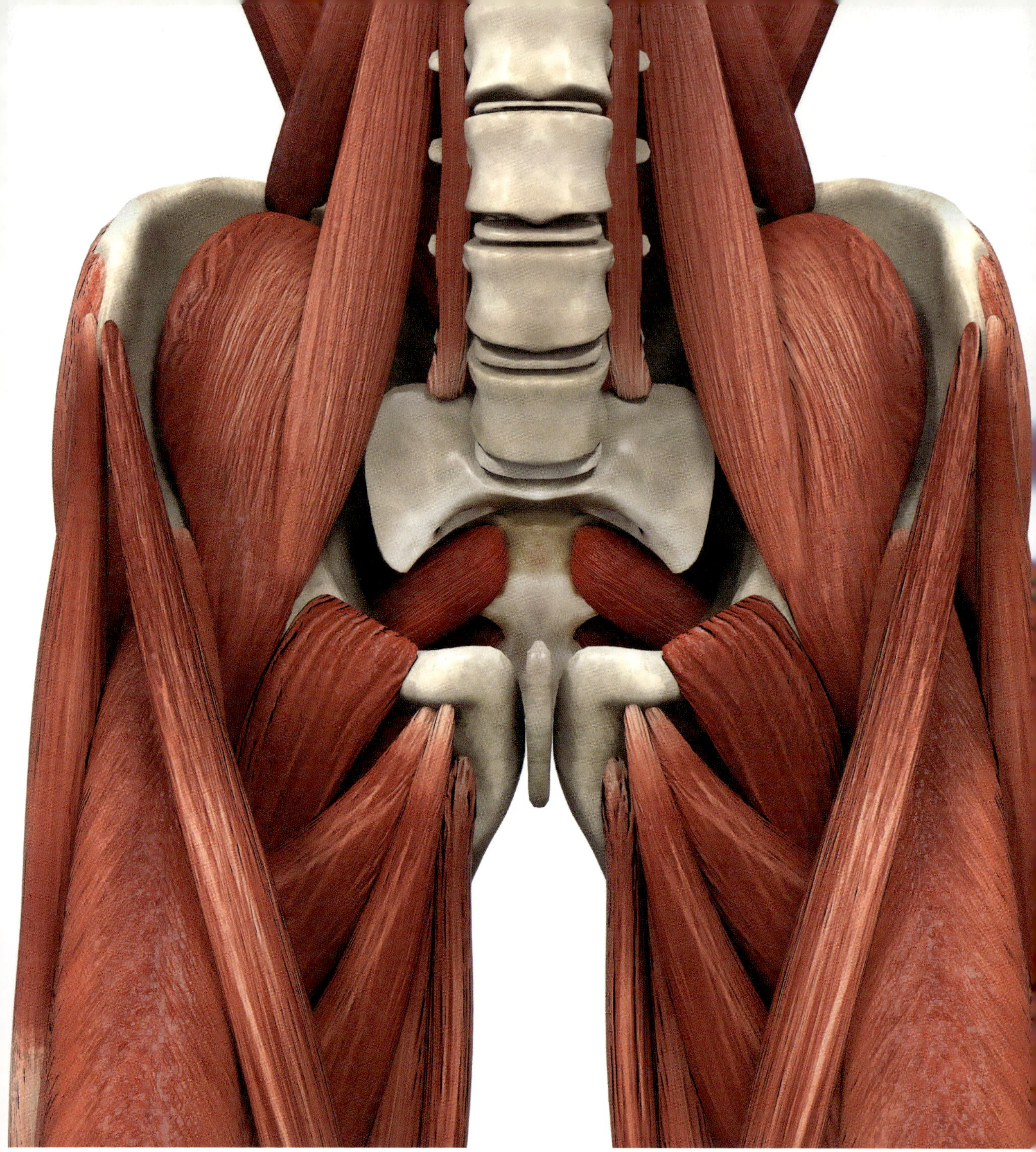

Your muscles are stretchy bands that move your bones by getting longer and shorter, a little like rubber bands.

Make Connections: What's a Safe Weight Workout?

So how much weight should you use? Experts say if you are able to lift 100 pounds, you should use 80 pounds and do 3 to 5 repetitions of each of 3–9 sets.

way to develop muscle strength. Using resistance bands is a good—and relatively inexpensive—way to train.

Many people like to build muscle strength by working with weights. Weight lifting can be effective. But it can also be dangerous. Using too much weight or lifting incorrectly can strain ***ligaments***, muscles, and ***tendons***. Working with someone knowledgeable can help keep you be safe. Experts recommend using lighter weights and doing more repetitions to get the biggest benefit.

Muscular Endurance

Muscular endurance refers to a muscle's ability to exert force without getting tired. Improving muscular endurance helps develop the muscles' slow-twitch fibers. These fibers handle low levels of force over a long period.

Endurance can be developed using the same activities as when improving cardiorespiratory endurance. These include jogging, swimming, and cycling.

Body Composition

You may know someone who looks small but weighs more than another person who has a larger body. Or two people who are the same height

Make Connections: The Problem with Falls

According to the Centers for Disease Control and Prevention (CDC), one out of three people over the age of 65 suffers a fall.

- Twenty to thirty percent of people who fall suffer cuts, hip fractures, or head traumas. Besides making it difficult to perform everyday tasks, these injuries can increase the risk of early death.
- Among the US population as a whole, falls are the most common cause of traumatic brain injuries (TBIs). In 2000, 46 percent of older adults who died from a fall did so because of TBIs caused by the fall.
- Even if someone who falls is not physically injured, she may become afraid of falling again. So instead of being active, she may limit her activities. While understandable, it has long-term effects. Lack of activity can lead to more flexibility problems and a decrease in physical fitness.

and have the same waist measurement but weigh different amounts. This is because of body composition. Body composition refers to the muscle, bone, and fat makeup of a person's body. It is also called the muscle-bone-fat ratio.

Some people mistakenly think muscle weighs more than fat. No matter what one is weighing, a pound will always equal 16 ounces; "A pound is a pound the world around." But muscle is denser than fat and takes up less room in the body. When measured in terms of volume, muscle weighs more per cubic inch than fat. So if measuring by volume, muscle does weigh more. This is why body size can be misleading in terms of how much someone weighs.

Flexibility

Flexibility describes the ability of a joint to move. Joints are what allow your body to move. Without them, you'd be just a straight column unable to bend. Imagine trying to walk if your knees wouldn't bend—or throw a ball if your elbows and shoulders were straight and solid! If your joints have a good range of motion—in other words, if you are flexible—you can move easily. You can combine movements without a problem. This means you can walk more smoothly, for example.

Flexibility can decrease as you age. When this happens, walking, for instance, may become difficult. Someone with flexibility issues may stumble. For people without flexibility problems, a crack in the sidewalk or walking on an uneven surface will likely not cause any problems. But if a person has limited flexibility, he may be unable to move his feet to avoid falling.

Besides the risk of falling, lack of mobility can be very painful. Arthritis is a condition that makes joints stiff, sore, and achy. Maintaining flexibility throughout your life can help delay some forms of arthritis, and it can lessen the painful effects if you do develop the condition.

As with most areas of fitness, you can start today doing things that will lessen the chances of developing a condition that will threaten your flexibility in the future. Activities that stretch your muscles help improve flexibility. Try swimming, or do some yoga.

THE ROLE OF FOOD IN FITNESS

You get in the car with your mom to go to the mall. The two of you are chatting about school, friends, and where at the mall you will have lunch. It's a good day. But then the car slows down. Mom presses on the accelerator, but the car doesn't go any faster. In fact, it slows down even more. Finally, you can't hear the motor at all, and your mother steers over to the side of the road just as the car comes to a stop. You look over at the dashboard, and the reason the car stopped is clear. The gas gauge is on E. Yup, the car is out of gas. Someone forgot to fill the gas tank.

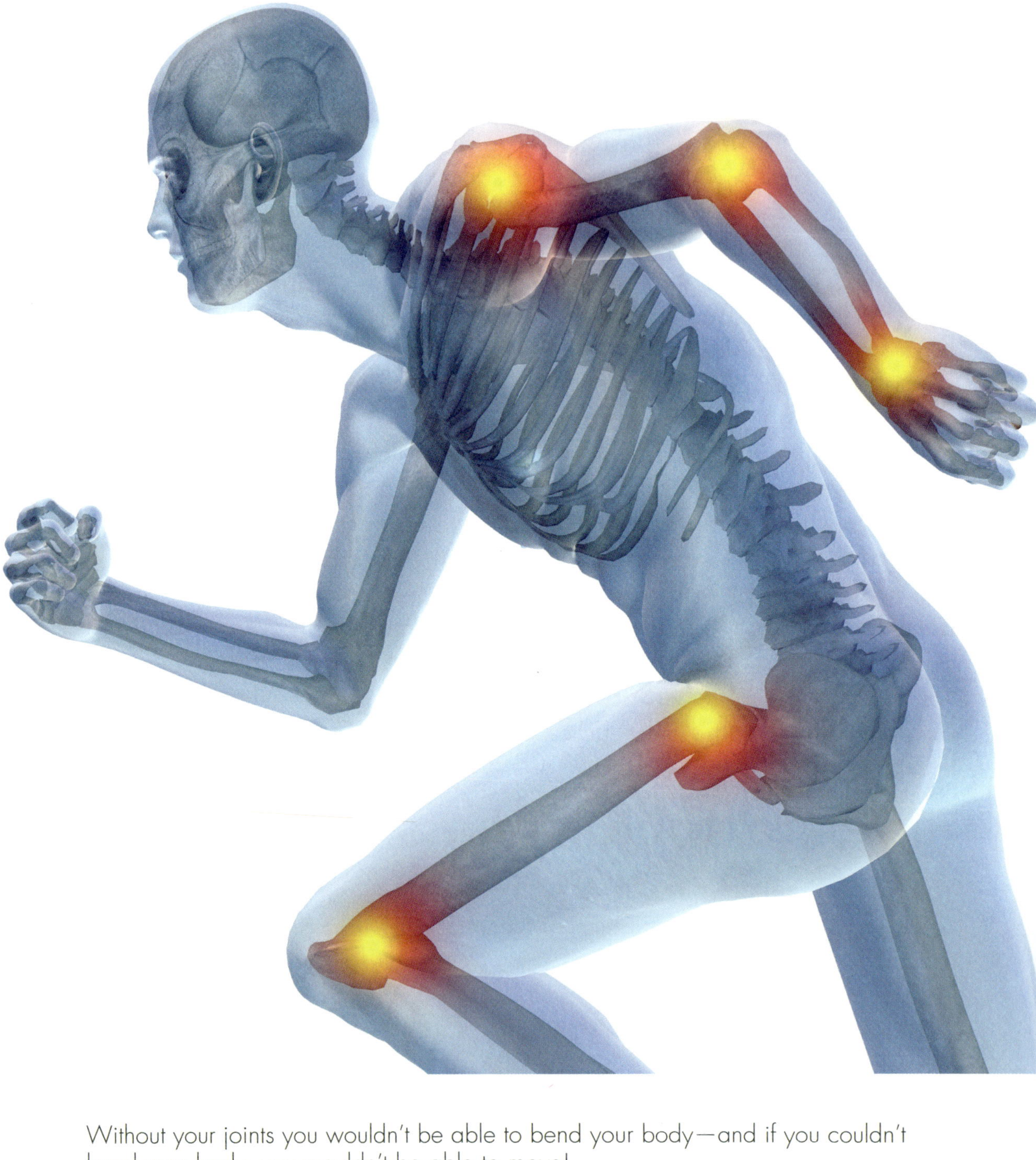

Without your joints you wouldn't be able to bend your body—and if you couldn't bend your body, you wouldn't be able to move!

Your body is like that car. It won't run without fuel. The car gets its fuel from gasoline, but your body's fuel comes from the energy you take in through food. Food provides energy in calories. A calorie is a unit of measurement. It's used to measure how much energy foods will produce in the body.

The type of calories you put into your body is important. Your body needs to take in the ***nutrients*** it needs, in the amounts it needs, to be fit. The nutrients the body needs can be divided into groups.

Carbohydrates

When your body needs energy, the first things it looks for are carbohydrates, which make glucose. They help send energy to all parts of the body.

There are simple and complex carbohydrates. Simple carbohydrates are found in many ***processed*** foods. Soda and candy often contain large amounts of simple carbohydrates, usually in the form of sugar, which provide the body with quick energy. But the energy does not last long. There is a quick burst, and then you might "crash" when the effect over.

Complex carbohydrates can be found in less-processed foods, including whole grains. It takes longer for the body to feel the effects of complex carbohydrates, but they last longer in the body. Complex carbohydrates provide more nutrition.

When you do not take in enough carbohydrates, the body makes the glucose it needs from protein. If you consume too many carbohydrates, your body converts them to fat to store for future needs.

Protein

Protein also comes from what you eat. Your body breaks down the protein into amino acids. The body uses these amino acids to build and repair parts of your body. Your body needs a lot of protein to support and build muscles. The immune system also uses protein for to make the chemicals it needs. The nervous system and organs use protein too.

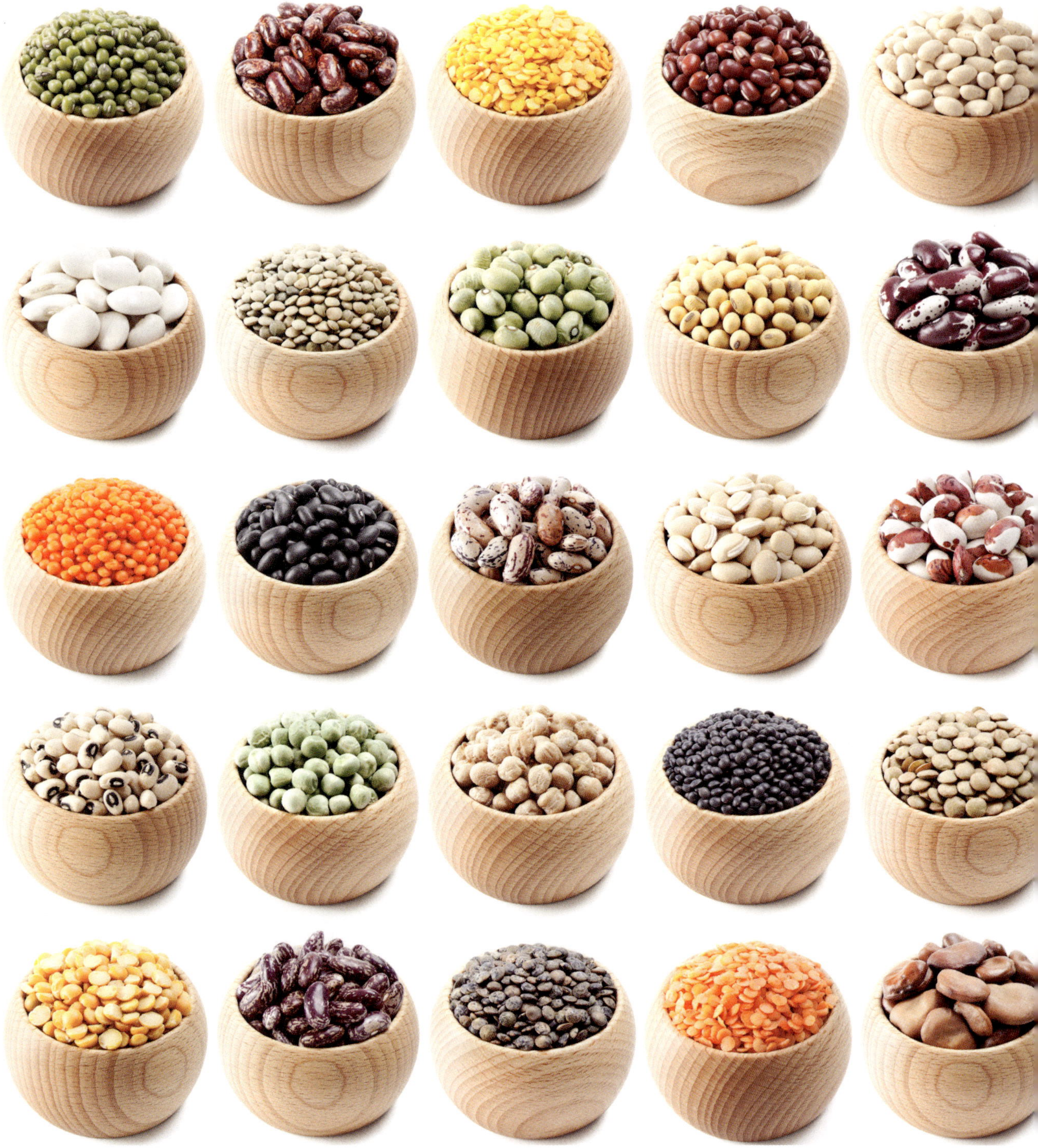

These are all different kinds of legumes, all of which are good sources of protein.

Many people do not eat meat because of health, philosophical, or religious reasons. For those people, it is important to find other sources of protein, such as ***legumes*** and dairy foods.

Fats

Despite the bad publicity fats get, they are necessary for good health. Fat is contained in membranes that surrounds the cells in your body. Your brain needs fatty acids. And fats are needed to signal hormone production and release.

Like carbohydrates, there are different types of fats. Monosaturated fats are the healthiest, and trans-fats are generally considered the unhealthiest. (Types of fats are discussed more in chapter 2.)

Vitamins and Minerals

The body needs large amounts of carbohydrates, protein, and fats. But the body also needs small amounts of vitamins and minerals to be healthy, function efficiently, and be fit. Vitamins and minerals' main purposes are generally to help a chemical reaction happen more quickly and efficiently. For example, when you consume something containing vitamin B, carbohydrates are burned more quickly, providing you with more energy. Vitamin A, found in carrots, helps with vision, the vitamin C you get in oranges and many other foods helps your immune system stay strong, and zinc is involved in many ***metabolic*** processes. Calcium is the most plentiful mineral in the body. It is found in many foods, including milk, cheese, almonds, and kale. Calcium helps keep your bones and teeth strong.

Antioxidants

The sun, pollution, and smoke have negative effects on the body's cells. Sometime people compare their effects to the rusting of metal, where metal breaks down as it combines with oxygen. That's not exactly what happens inside your body, of course, but certain kinds of oxygen can cause damage to your body's cells. Consuming antioxidants, although

4. What is the difference between simple carbohydrates and complex carbohydrates?
5. List two nonmeat sources of protein.

Vegetables and fruits are good sources of minerals and vitamins. Can you recognize the vegetables and fruits shown here?

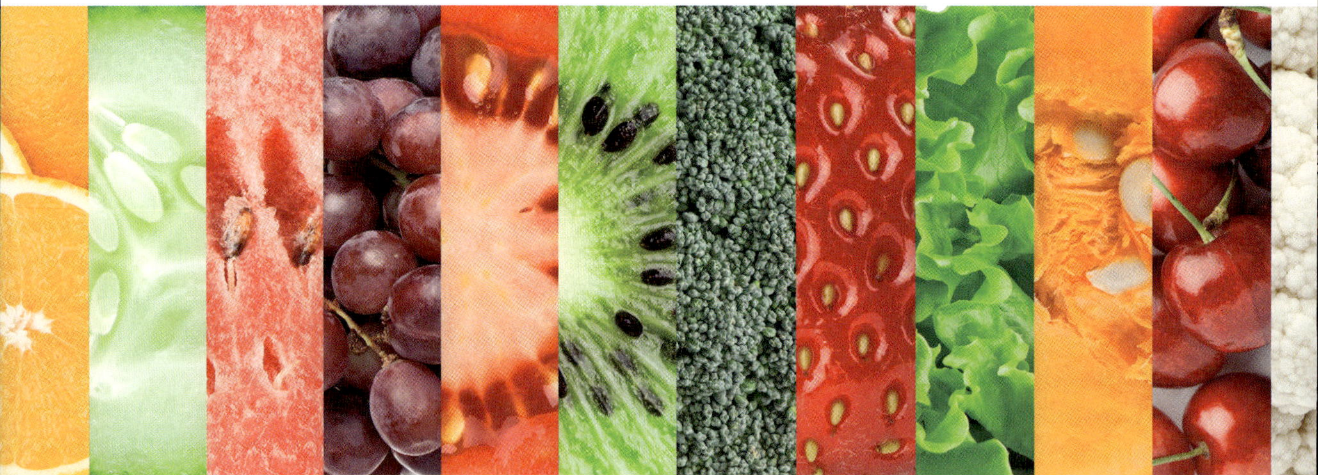

Answer: From left to right, oranges, cucumber, watermelon, grapes, tomato, kiwi fruit, broccoli, strawberry, lettuce, squash, cherries, cauliflower.

Research Project

This chapter gives a list of things that make up physical fitness. Using the information provided in this chapter, as well as information you find on the Internet or in the library, compile a list of activities you can do now to get physically fit or stay fit. Keep in mind conditions you want to avoid, if possible, in the future.

not necessary for fitness, can help delay and prevent those effects on the body.

Antioxidants are found in phytochemicals of fruits and vegetables, as well as from other sources. Red beans, red apples, blueberries, and cranberries are all good sources of antioxidants.

Knowing as much as you can about the nutrients in foods can help you make the right choices to keep you healthy for a lifetime.

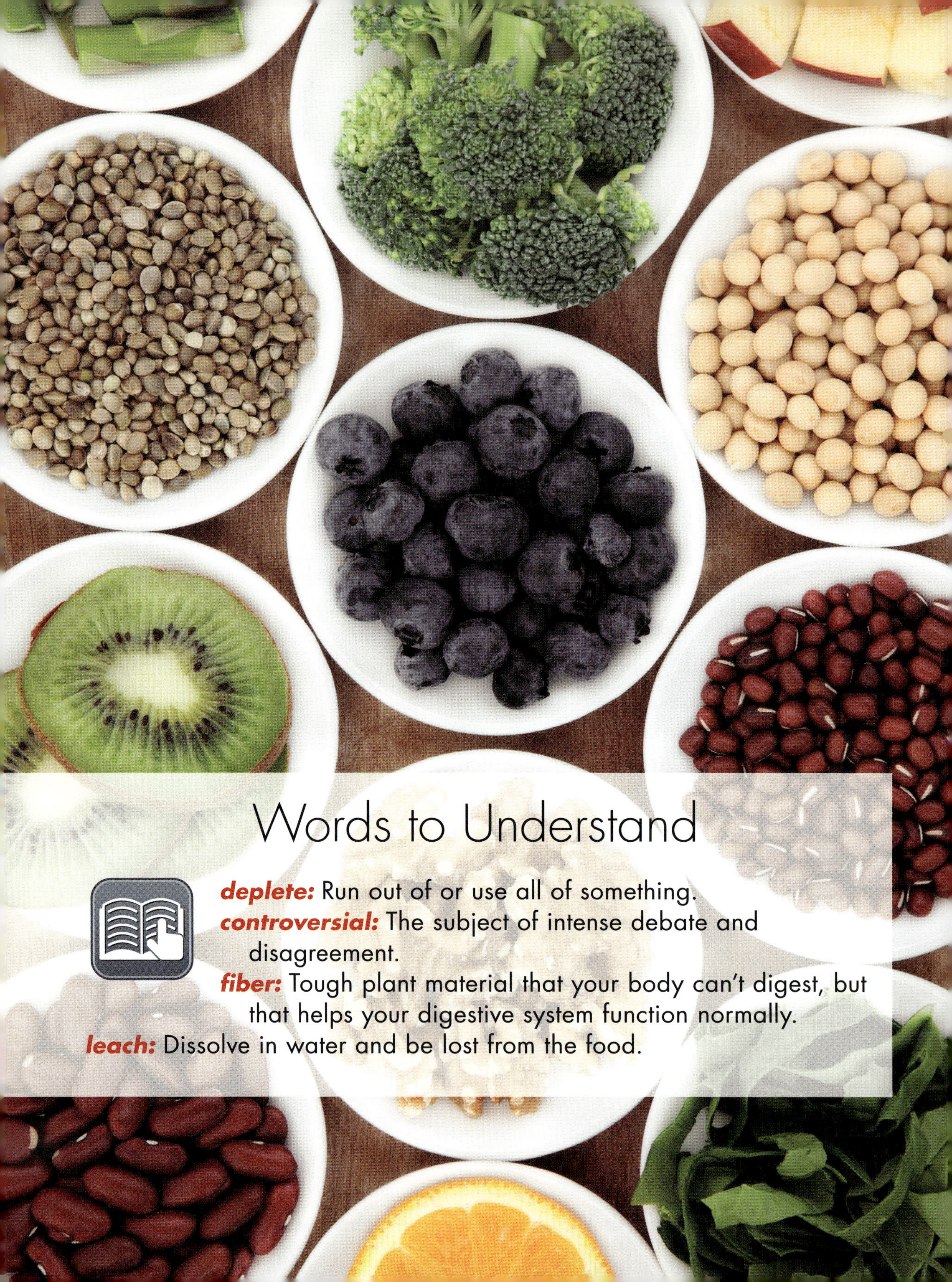

Words to Understand

deplete: Run out of or use all of something.

controversial: The subject of intense debate and disagreement.

fiber: Tough plant material that your body can't digest, but that helps your digestive system function normally.

leach: Dissolve in water and be lost from the food.

Chapter Two

Foods to Eat, Foods to Avoid

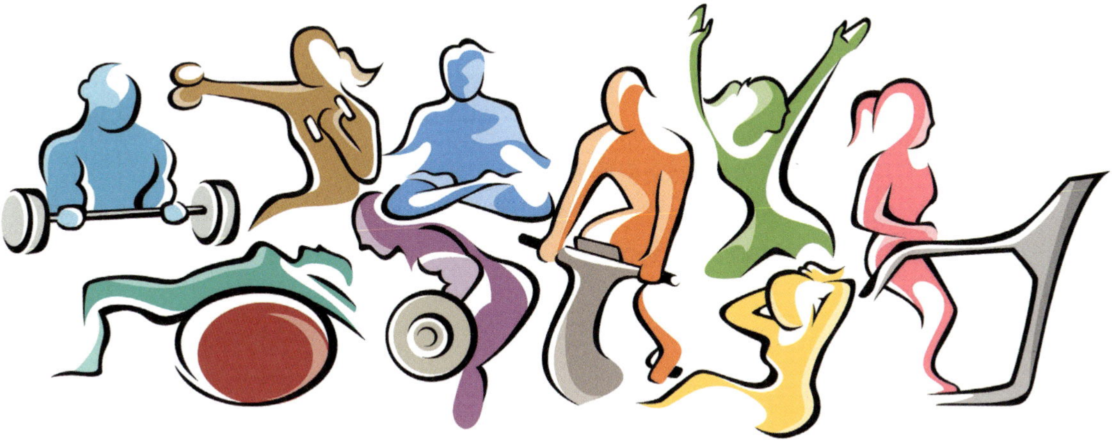

Knowing the right foods to eat for fitness can be difficult. After all, there are a lot of foods to choose from. To help us make informed food choices, the US Department of Agriculture (USDA) has divided foods into five groups.

VEGETABLES

Vegetables are good sources of iron, vitamin B, and other nutrients. Although most vegetables are grown in the ground, hydroponic vegetable growing, where plants are grown in water, is becoming increasingly popular. There is a wide variety of vegetables to choose from. Greens, tomatoes, cucumbers, green beans, broccoli—the list seems to go on and on.

The vegetable category has good and better choices. For example, sweet potatoes have slightly more nutritional value than white potatoes. They both contain potassium, with sweet potatoes having a slight advantage. Sweet potatoes have much more beta carotene. The body converts beta carotene to vitamin A, which benefits vision and other things.

FRUITS

Fruits contain many of the same nutrients found in vegetables. They are a great source of vitamin C. Blueberries and cranberries are among the fruits containing high levels of antioxidants. Cranberries and cranberry juice have long been used to prevent urinary tract infections.

Cooking can ***deplete*** some of a food's nutrients. Because they are usually eaten raw, fruits hold on to their nutrients. This means the body can have the benefits of more of fruits' nutritional benefits.

Most fruits are sweet. This sweetness attracts many people to fruit. And while getting people to eat fruit is a good thing, the sweetness can be problematic to some people, including those with diabetes. Among the fruits with the highest sugar levels are tangerines, cherries, grapes, pomegranates, mangoes, figs, and bananas. Dried fruit, like raisins and prunes, also contain a lot of sugar. Substitute less-sweet fruits—like lemons, most berries, and melons—for fruits high in sugar.

GRAINS

Grains are the seeds of grass plants. They are also referred to as cereal grains. Rice, wheat, oats, barley, quinoa, and corn are among the most common grains. Most people eat grains every day.

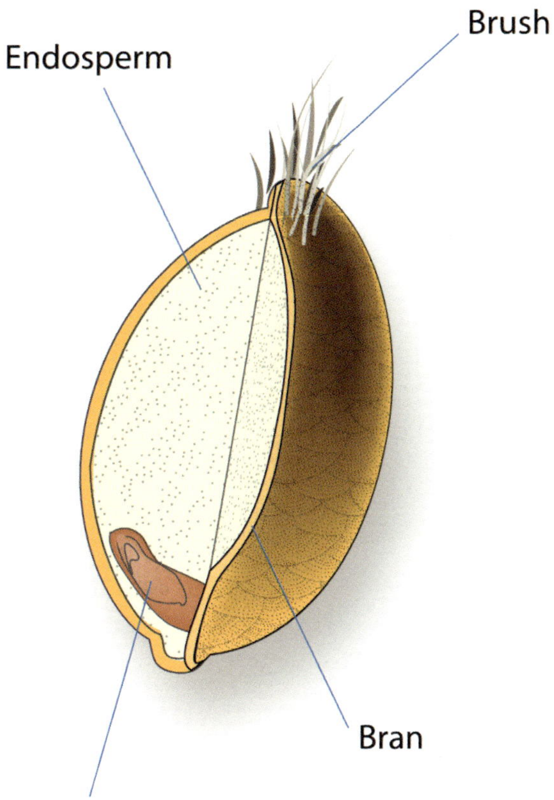

A Wheat Kernel

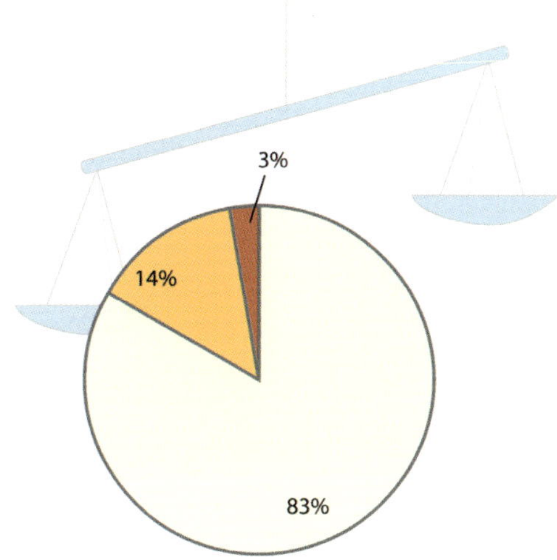

Composition by weight

	Carb./g	Protein/g	Fat/g	Fiber/g	Iron (% daily req.)	Others
Bran	63	16	3	43	59	vitamin Bs
Endosperm	79	7	0	4	7	
Germ	52	23	10	14	35	vitamin Bs omega-3/6 lipids

Nutritional Value (per 100g)

This diagram shows the parts of a grain of a wheat, with the nutritional values of each. As you can see, most of the grain's nutrients are found in the bran and germ.

Make Connections: Plant-Based Protein

Some people cannot or choose not to eat meat or meat products. As an alternative to eating meat-based protein, they can turn to several plant-based options. They include:

- quinoa
- hemp seeds
- chia seeds
- beans
- peas
- asparagus
- pumpkin seeds
- broccoli
- lentils
- sunflower seeds

There are whole grains and refined grains. Seeds contain germ, endosperm, and bran. Whole grains contain all of those elements. Refined grains contain only the endosperm. Whenever possible, eat mostly products made from whole grains. They are more nutritious and contain complex carbohydrates rather than simple ones.

Some people have an allergy or sensitivity to wheat, usually to the gluten contained in wheat. This can cause problems when it comes to foods we eat every day, like bread and pasta. Today there are increasing numbers of products available for people with these sensitivities. Wheat flour is often replaced with flour made from rice or oats.

PROTEINS

When we hear the word "protein," the first thing that probably comes to mind is meat. While meat is a major source of protein, many other foods also contain protein. These include eggs, beans, and nuts.

Besides protein, many meats contain a significant amount of fat. Not everyone wants that fat in their diet. Leaner cuts of beef can be found in

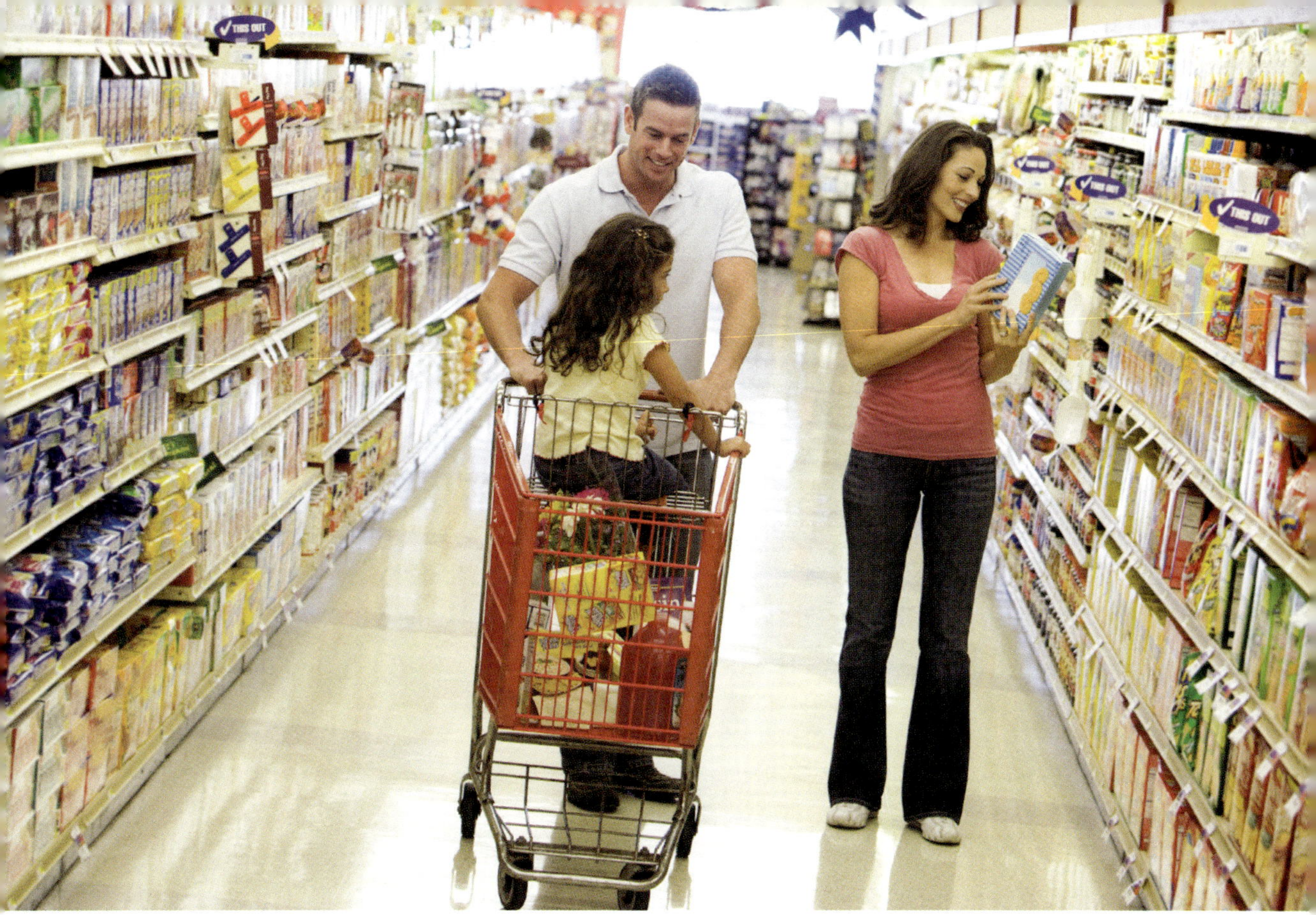

Grocery stores are full of packaged foods. They're convenient and they stay fresh on the shelves—but they're often not as nutritious as whole foods.

almost every grocery store. Chicken and turkey have lower amounts of fat. You can also use other sources of protein and avoid the issue of fat.

DAIRY

To be considered a dairy food, the food must come from mammals' milk. Milk, yogurt, and cheese are dairy foods. In the United States, most milk comes from cows, but goat milk is also used to produce dairy products.

Dairy products contain vitamin D and calcium. For many people, these sources are the primary sources for these important nutrients.

Unfortunately, people who are lactose intolerant cannot drink milk or eat dairy food. Their bodies cannot digest lactose, a type of sugar found in milk and milk products. If they consume something containing milk, people who are lactose intolerant can have extreme pain and diarrhea, among other symptoms. People who cannot have milk need to use other calcium and vitamin D sources, including dark-green, leafy vegetables. For some, goat milk is an option.

Another option for those with lactose intolerance—or those who simply want a healthier food—are cultured dairy products. Among them are butter, buttermilk, yogurt, and some aged cheeses. In production, beneficial bacteria are added to the milk. They turn most of the lactose into lactic acid, which makes the milk easier to digest.

FATS

Though not considered a food group using the FDA's current nutritional recommendations, fats play an important role in health and fitness. They are essential to digestion. But not all fats are created equal.

Fats are composed of fatty acids. These fatty acids are categorized based on their chemical makeup. All have carbon atoms surrounded by hydrogen atoms. A a fat molecule with no double bonds between carbon atoms is a *saturated fat,* such as the fat found in beef. A fat with double bonds in it is an *unsaturated fat.* Unsaturated fat is found in olive oil and lard. If only one pair of carbon atoms is connected with a double bond, we have *monosaturated fat. Polyunsaturated fat* occurs when a fat molecule has two or more double bonds between carbon atoms. This is the type of fat found in corn oil.

Many of the fats we eat today are hydrogenated, meaning they were made using unsaturated oil. Partially hydrogenated fats, also called trans fats, have had an atom added to an unsaturated fat. When a food contains trans fats, it has a longer shelf life. But research has also shown trans fats can raise bad cholesterol levels and potentially cause some kinds of cancer. In late 2013, the FDA announced it was taking steps to ban trans fats.

Fat intake is one of the most ***controversial*** food-related topics.

Few nutrition experts dispute the health benefits of a fatty acid called omega 3, found in fish. Whether it is better to eat animal-derived or plant-derived fats is still debated.

WHOLE OR PROCESSED?

There are a plenty of other food debates. Whole foods—or processed? That's another hot topic in the nutrition world.

You're probably more familiar with processed foods, though you might not know it. Food scientists engineered much of the food found in supermarkets; it's been manufactured, like any other object you might buy at a store. In the 1920s, dentist Weston A. Price found many of his patients were experiencing a serious decline in their health. He researched the phenomenon and discovered healthy people all over the world had some things in common. They didn't eat refined sugar, white flour, or mass-produced canned foods. They didn't use vegetable oils. And this population also had low instances of heart disease, diabetes, or cancer—all common during Price's time and even more so today. Price also found that the healthier people ate vitamin- and mineral-rich foods, animal fats (including butter), and organ meats. Much of their diet was fermented (think sauerkraut, pickles, and yogurt) or eaten raw.

Today, this is not the case for most of us. We go to the supermarket and find hundreds of canned foods, frozen dinners, and other already-prepared products. It's easy to see their attraction. After all, most of us lead busy lives. Without such conveniences, we might give in to the temptation of a quick run to a drive-through, and we all know how bad that food can be. But are those convenience foods any better? In many cases, no. They often contain highly processed ingredients. Look at the labels. Do you know what those ingredients are or why they've been included? Can you pronounce them? Many of these odd-sounding things help preserve food, so that the food won't spoil or get stale.

And how many ingredients are there? Take bread, for example. If you want to make basic bread, you need four ingredients: flour, salt, water, and yeast. The label for a store-bought bread can have twenty ingredients—if not more! In some cases, the ingredients include added

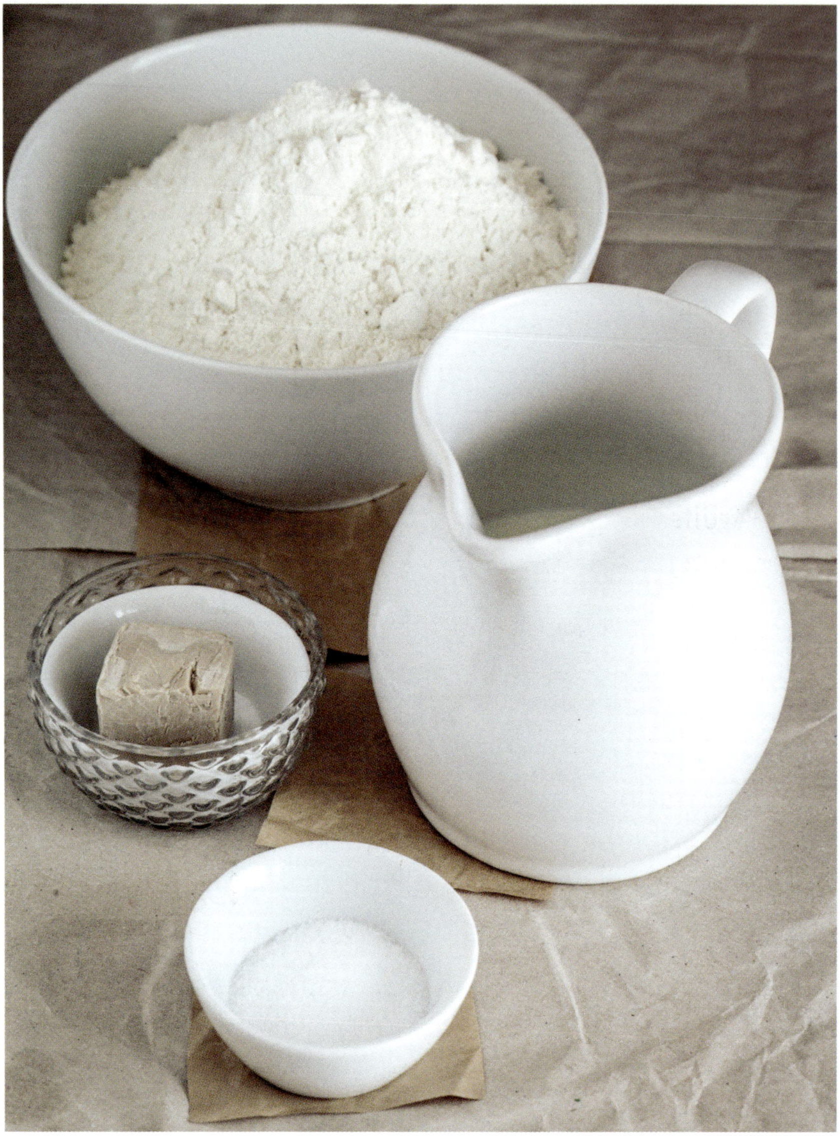

These are all the ingredients you need to make bread from scratch (above). Now compare that to this ingredients label from a package of store-bought bread (below).

INGREDIENTS: Enriched Wheat Flour(Unbleached Wheat Flour, Malted Barley Flour, Niacin, Reduced Iron, Potassium Bromate, Thiamine Mononitrate, Riboflavin, Folic Acid), Water, Vegetable Shortening (Partially Hydrogenated Soybean and Cottonseed Oils,Soybean Oil, Soybean Lecithin with Mono- and Diglycerides, Vitamin A Palmitate), Butter, Sugar, Contains 2% or less of: Leavening(Yeast, Baking Powder [Sodium Bicarbonate, Cornstarch, Sodium Aluminum Phosphate, Calcium Sulfate, Monocalcium Phosphate]), Non-Fat Dry Milk, Salt, Dough Conditioner (Wheat Flour, DATEM, Dextrose, Soybean Oil, Ascorbic Acid, L-Cysteine, Azodicarbonamide(ADA), Calcium Stearoyl-2 Lactylate, Enzymes), Eggs, Artificial Flavor, Preservatives(Calcium Propionate, Potassium Sorbate, Citric Acid).

nutrients. Why would factories add nutrients, though? One reason is because refined, processed flour has lost most of its nutrients.

Whole foods are ones that are as close to their natural form as possible and as least-processed as possible. Many health experts believe the best way to be healthy and fit is to eat more whole foods. Whole foods keep their ***fiber***, as well the nutrients that are good for us, which are often removed in processed foods.

But how can you add more whole foods to your diet? On your next trip to the grocery store, spend most of your time shopping in the outer aisles. That's where you're more likely to find whole, healthier foods. Pick up fresh fruits, vegetables, and beans. They are great sources of fiber and vitamins. When possible, buy whole-grain versions of foods, including bread and pasta. Like chicken or fish nuggets? That's okay, but make them yourself. Cut a chicken breast or piece of fish into cubes and cook. That way, you will know you're getting whole pieces of chicken or fish. You won't need to wonder if there is anything else in the ground meat or fish that was reshaped to create nuggets.

But what if you want some fruits or vegetables that aren't available in the store's produce department? You don't have to go without—just skip the temptation to pick up a can. Instead, check out the frozen-food aisle. Most frozen vegetables and fruits are flash frozen after being picked, locking nutrition into the frozen fruits or vegetables. They make good substitutes when fresh ones aren't available. Just be sure to read the label on the package to make sure it doesn't include other things, such as sugar or syrup.

ORGANIC FOODS

Over the years, the variety of organic foods available in our supermarkets has increased. And that's just in the fresh food sections! But do we need to buy organic to be healthy?

It depends on whom you ask. Some food experts say using the word "organic" is just a marketing trick so stores can charge more. Others claim you that organic foods really are healthier. The truth probably lies somewhere in the middle.

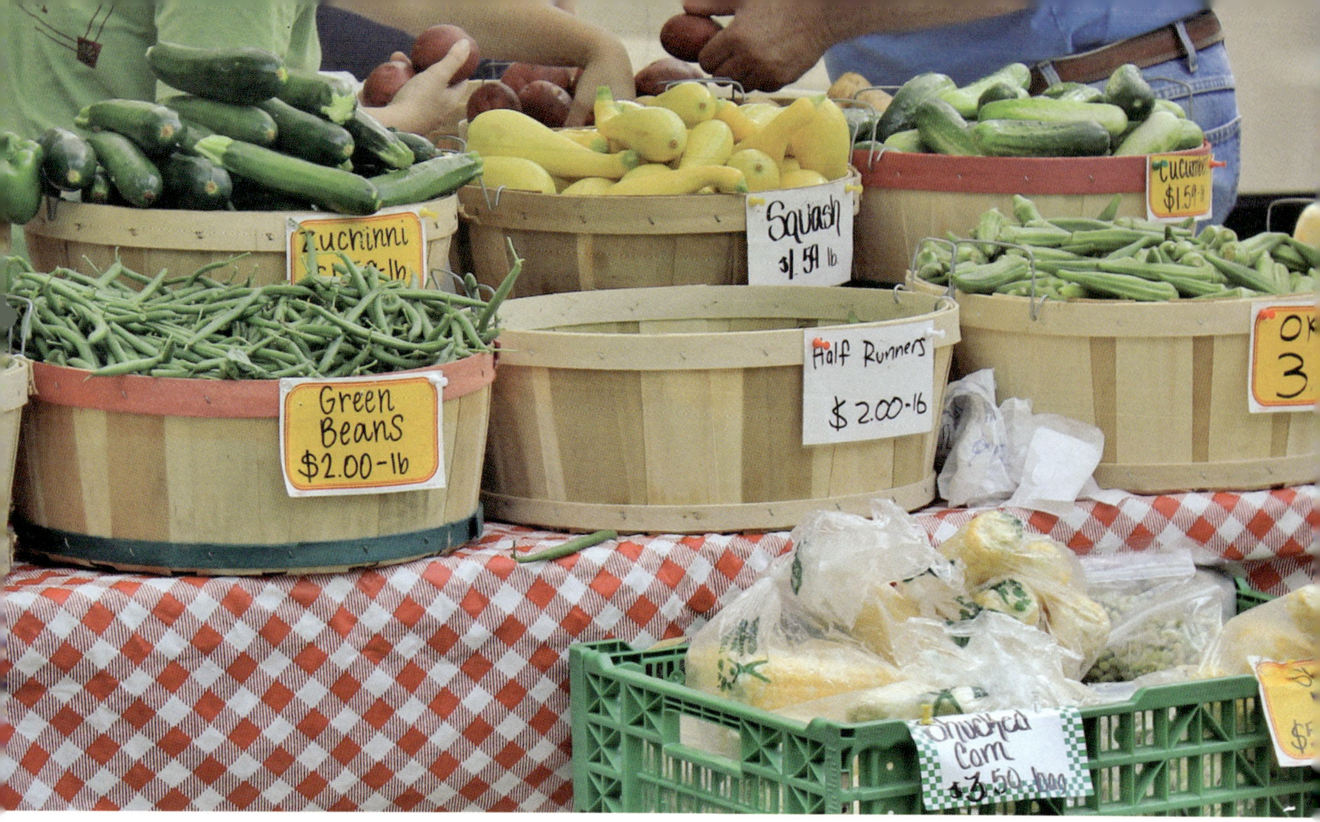

You can be sure that the food you buy at a farmer's market is fresh. You also know that it didn't have to travel far to reach you.

What Does Organic Mean?

Organic foods are grown or raised without the use of pesticides (chemicals used to kill insects and other pests), synthetic fertilizers (chemicals added to the soil to make plants grow better), sewage sludge (the solid material left after water is removed from the waste that comes from toilets), genetically modified organisms (plants or animals that have been specially designed by scientists to have certain traits), or ionizing radiation (zaps of high-energy waves that change the molecules of a plant or food product). None of those things sound particularly appealing, do they? Also, in order to be labeled organic, animals that produce meat, eggs, or dairy products cannot take antibiotics or growth hormones.

The USDA oversees the National Organic Program (NOP), which defines organic. If farmers or ranchers want their products to carry the "organic" label, a government-approved inspector visits the farms or ranches to make sure they are following all the NOP rules. Any processors that handle the food before it gets to the grocery store must be certified as well.

It takes time to meet all the NOP requirements—and it's expensive. Many food producers choose to forgo the certification program. Though they cannot claim to be organic, they can say their food is grown or raised in an *organic manner*. It's up to consumers to decide if they want to purchase such products.

The Dirty Dozen

But do we need to buy organic food? It's a personal decision. Being fit probably doesn't require buying and eating organic food. On the other hand, consuming organic food can help make sure you're only getting what you want. It lessens the worry caused by wondering what long-term effects a particular fertilizer or pesticide can have on your body.

Most food experts believe it is not necessary to buy organic versions of all foods. After all, they do generally cost more. According to Organic.com, there are twelve foods, however, that are more likely to be contaminated if they're not organic:

- peaches
- apples
- bell peppers
- celery
- nectarines
- strawberries
- cherries
- pears
- imported grapes
- spinach

Make Connections

Read the label. Go beyond information regarding fat grams, sugar content, serving size, and calorie count. Pay attention to the ingredients. The more ingredients in a product, the more likely it has been extensively processed.

Eat more whole foods. As you eat foods that are packed with nutrients, you may find yourself actually eating less.

Choose whole grains. But again, read the label. It may say "whole grain" on the package, and it may have that whole-grain "look" you expect in healthy products. Sometimes, however, things aren't as they seem. Some whole-grain products contain white flour and other ingredients you may be trying to avoid.

Be a regular at the farmers' market or locavore store. You'll be able to pick up fresh, seasonal, locally grown food. Most have regulations about how far the produce and other foods are allowed to travel before reaching the market.

Start a garden. An amazing amount of food can be grown in a small space. Purchase some organic seeds and organic soil and plant a small garden plot or use containers. Then save the seeds from your crop to plant the following year. To learn about growing in limited space, check out the *Square Foot Gardening Foundation* (squarefootgardening.org/square-foot-gardening-method).

- lettuce
- potatoes

On the other hand, some foods are not likely to be contaminated. If you're looking to budget the grocery money you spend on organic

Text-Dependent Questions

1. What are some of the healthy things in vegetables?
2. Explain the health benefits of eating whole grains.
3. How does the author define "whole foods"?
4. The author lists the "Dirty Dozen" of foods. What makes them "dirty"?
5. Describe five ways to have a more healthy diet, as listed in the sidebar.

foods, you can save by buying regular types of these vegetables and fruits:

- onions
- avocados
- frozen sweet corn
- pineapples
- mangoes
- asparagus
- frozen sweet peas
- kiwi fruit
- bananas
- cabbage
- broccoli
- papaya

HOW WE COOK

Eating to be fit extends beyond food choice to how we prepare our food. Boiling tends to cause foods to ***leach*** their nutrients into the liquid.

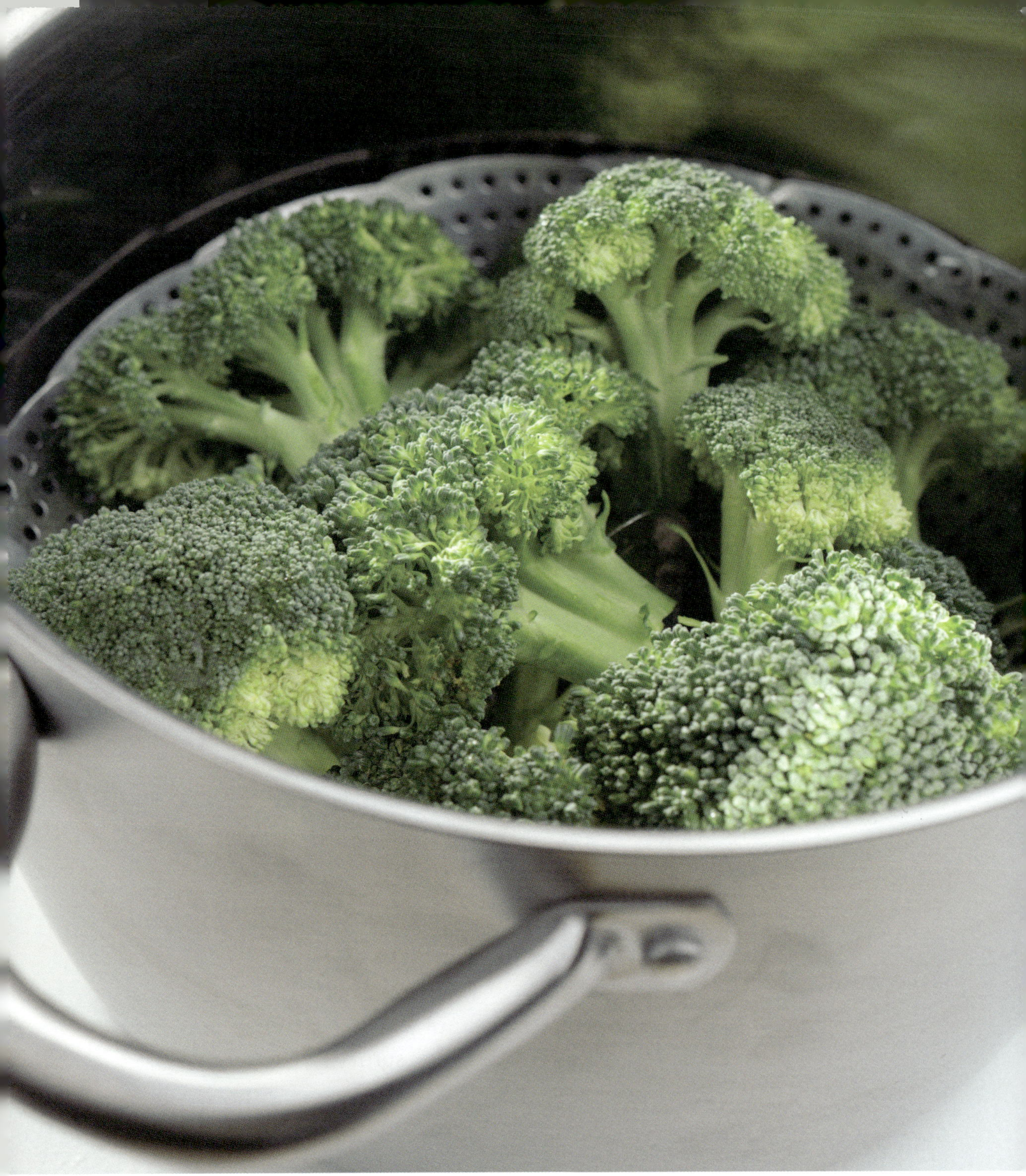

If you steam your broccoli instead of boil it, it will keep more of its nutrients.

Research Project

Using the information in this chapter and the newspaper insert with ads for the grocery store where your family shops, make a list of foods you can buy to keep you and your family healthy and fit. What organic foods would you put on the list, if any? Note what foods your family would usually buy. Should any of them be replaced to make your diet healthier?

This isn't a problem if you're making a soup or stew, and you're using the cooking liquid. But if you pour the liquid down the drain—well, there go a lot of nutrients.

Here are two other ways to avoid losing nutrition when preparing food:

- Steam foods. Contact with water is less, so nutrients are less likely to leach out of the food.
- Eat food raw. According to some experts, you should eat some raw fruits and vegetables every day.

Keep in mind, though, that cooking is not the only thing that causes fruit and vegetables to lose their nutritional value. Light and air also have negative effects. The best way to make sure you have fruits and vegetables at their best is to buy foods that are grown locally and that have been picked fairly recently. If you want to eat fruit and vegetables out of their normal harvest season, buy frozen ones.

Eating fresh, whole foods will go a long way to help you keep fit. But sometimes, it's not enough.

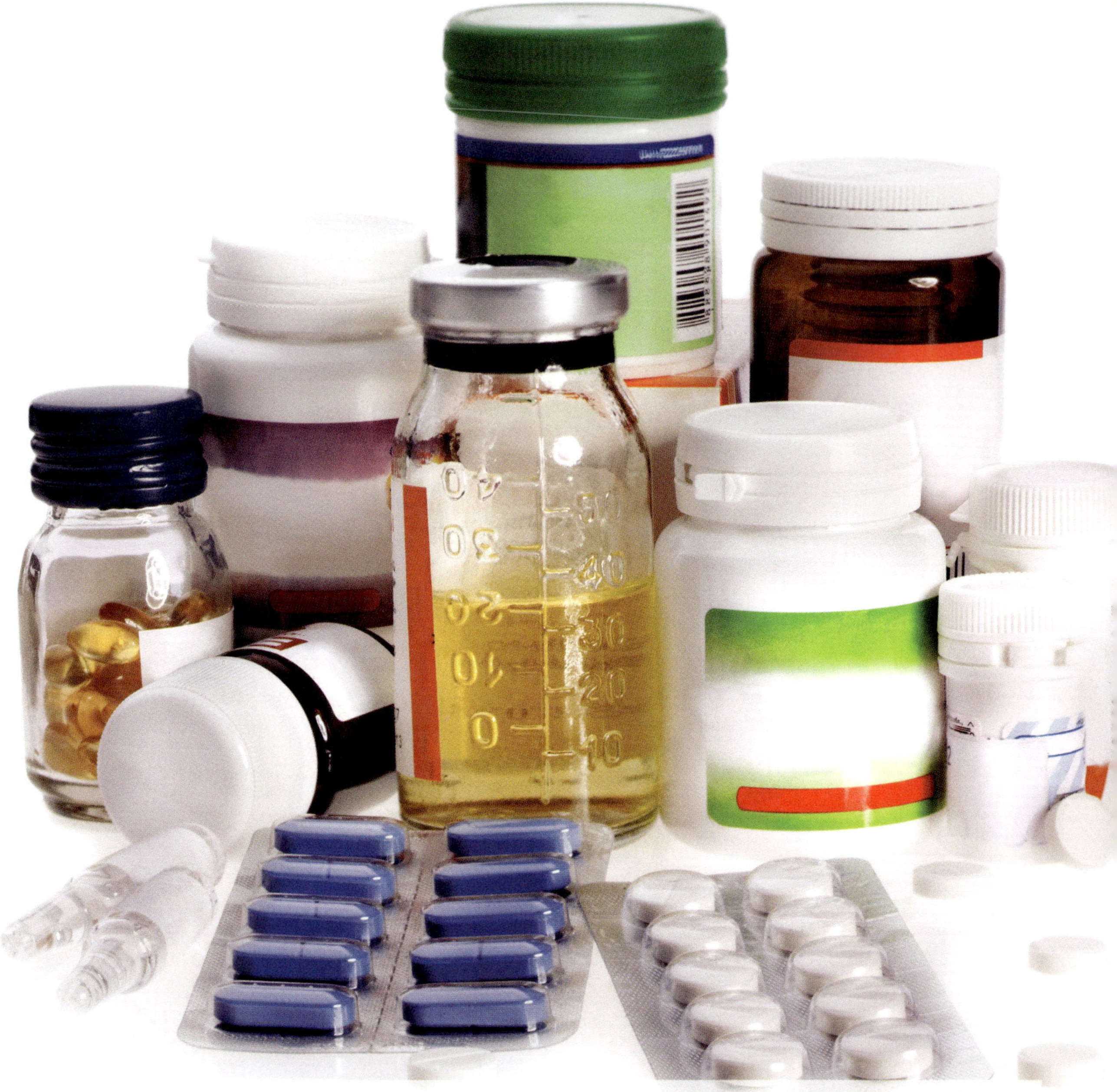

Words to Understand

regime: A program or plan for getting healthier.
synthesis: The process of creating something.

Chapter Three

Nutritional Supplements and Fitness

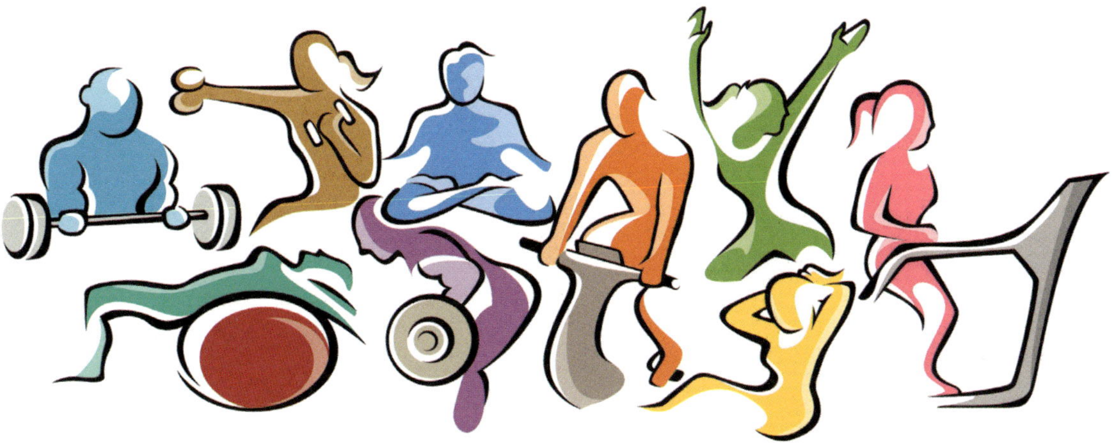

You and your friends are having lunch and talking. Each of you has brought a lunch from home. You know yours is healthy, because your family buys and eats healthy foods. You're not so sure about your friends'. But when you make a comment about their food choices—mostly junk food and packaged foods—they just shrug.

"I'm taking vitamin C," Stacy says.

"My dad makes me take a multivitamin," says Ian. "The kind that has minerals in it too."

Jennifer nods. "My parents shop at the health food store. They get all sorts of supplements that they make me take. My mom says that way she doesn't have to worry about whether I'm eating junk or not."

You look down at your lunch of whole-grain bread and tuna, with a dessert of fruit and yogurt. Then you give a shrug of your own. You like your lunch.

WHAT ARE NUTRITIONAL SUPPLEMENTS?

A healthy diet is the best way to get the nutrients you need. But sometimes nutritional supplements can help as well.

Nutritional supplements include vitamins and minerals, as well as pills and powders made from herbs and other plants. They are designed to provide you with things you are missing in your diet. Among the more common nutritional supplements are:

- acidophilus
- Echinacea
- fiber
- ginger
- glucosamine and/or chondroitin sulphate
- minerals
- omega-3 fatty acids
- St. John's wort
- saw palmetto
- vitamins

Multivitamins, pills containing more than one vitamin, are probably the most common supplements.

WHEN DO YOU NEED A SUPPLEMENT?

If you eat from the five food groups every day in the right amount (more on that in chapter 4), you probably do not need a supplement.

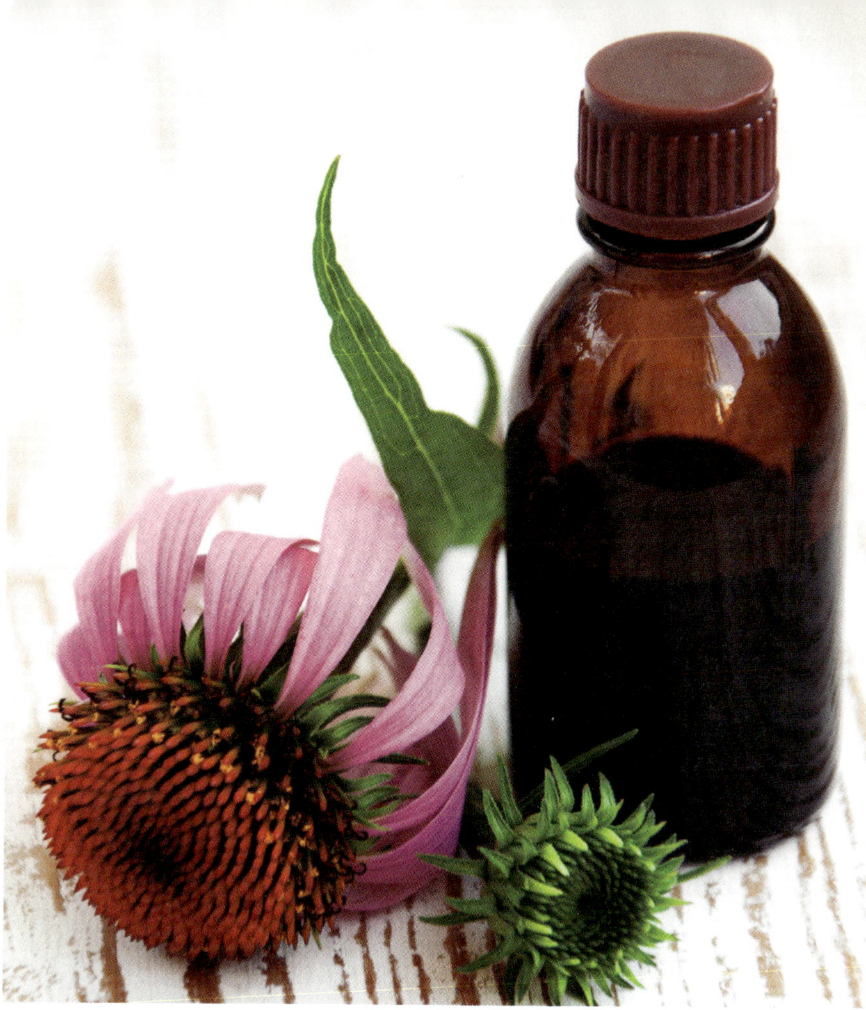

Echinacea is a supplement that comes from a flowering plant. Many people believe that taking it will help protect them against diseases, from the common cold to cancer. Scientific research has so far not found any evidence to support this.

But if you aren't eating a variety of foods, your body may lack vitamins and minerals. Though you may feel well now, your health and fitness may eventually suffer. Supplements can provide those missing nutrients. Keep in mind, though, that they are not meant to make up for not eating the right things.

Some people have physical conditions that mean they need to take nutritional supplements. People with pernicious anemia, for example, have a dangerously low supply of red blood cells. Your body needs vitamin B12 to create healthy red blood cells, but someone with pernicious anemia cannot absorb vitamin B12, so she cannot create the red

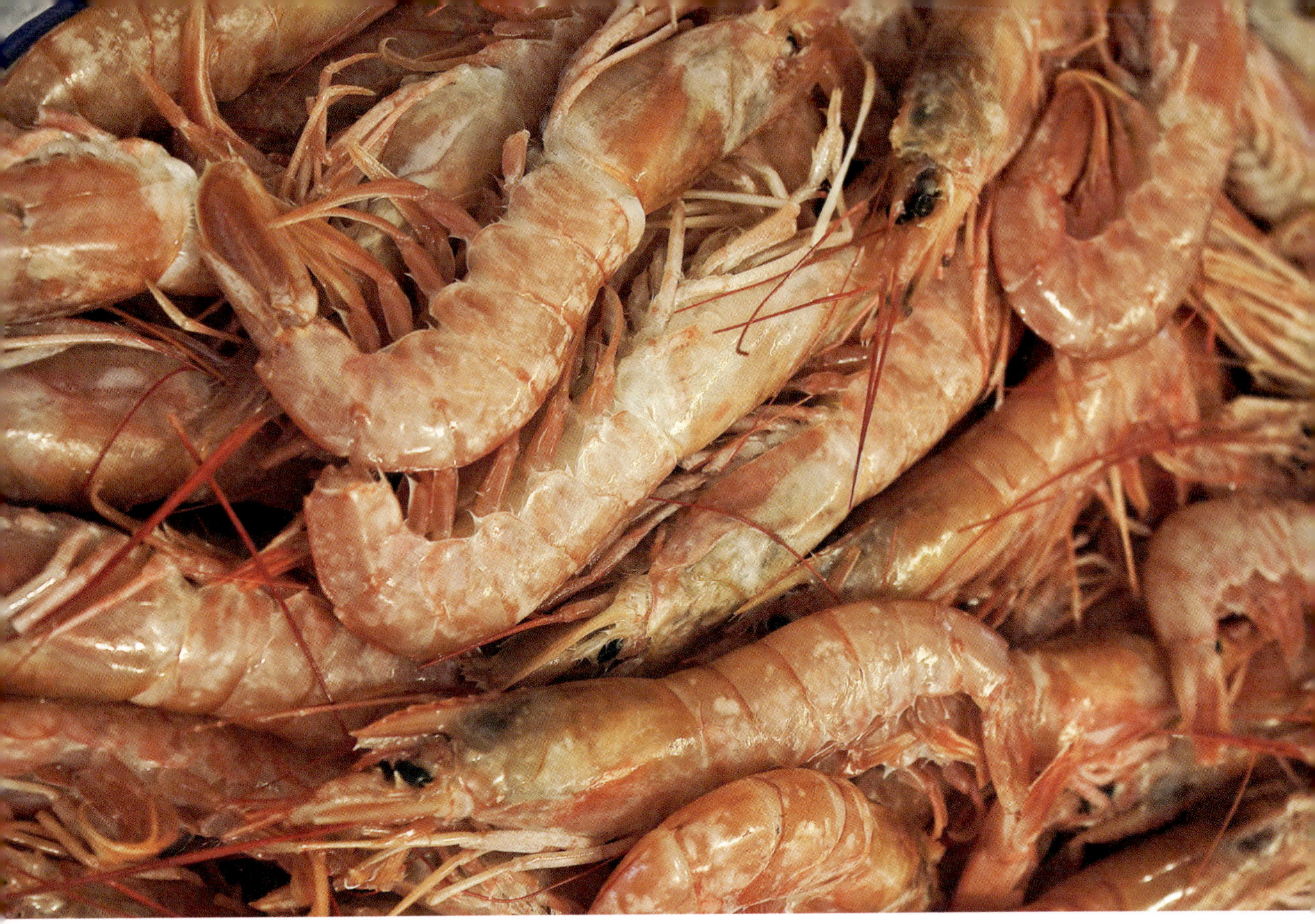

Glucosamine is a substance that's made from the shells of crustaceans like shrimp. There are claims that it may reduce joint pain—but research has yet to prove this.

blood cells her body needs. Without taking vitamin B12, her health is at risk.

Although nutritional supplements are sometimes used as part of a treatment ***regime***, don't try to treat yourself. Check with your health-care professional. She'll know if that is the proper course of action—assuming you really do have a medical condition.

ARE NUTRITIONAL SUPPLEMENTS SAFE?

Nutritional supplements are generally safe when taken as directed. However, you need to remember that they're not medicine. In the United States, the FDA carefully tests and approves all drugs—but when it

Nutritional Supplement Use on the Rise

An increasing number of children and teens are taking nutritional supplements. But many are not taking them because their diet lacks vitamins and minerals. According to a 2004 study, parents use dietary supplements to treat children with chronic health conditions, including cancer, cystic fibrosis, and attention-deficit/hyperactivity disorder. Some parents give their children with Down syndrome large doses of multivitamins. In most cases, there is no scientific evidence that these supplements work in the way that parents are hoping.

comes to supplements, it's all up to the supplements' manufacturers and distributors. Manufacturers and distributors are required to report any bad side effects, however, to the FDA. If a nutritional supplement is found to be unsafe after it goes on the market, the FDA can take it off the market.

Many supplements contain ingredients that could have strong effects on the body. This could make them unsafe in some situations and even damage your health. Among ways supplements can have bad—even fatal—effects is when:

- A person uses supplements with prescription or over-the-counter medication. The chemicals in the supplements can interact with the medicines in unpredictable ways. Some reactions can be life-threatening. If someone takes the prescription Coumadin, for example, as well as gingko, aspirin, or vitamin E, his blood may become dangerously thin.

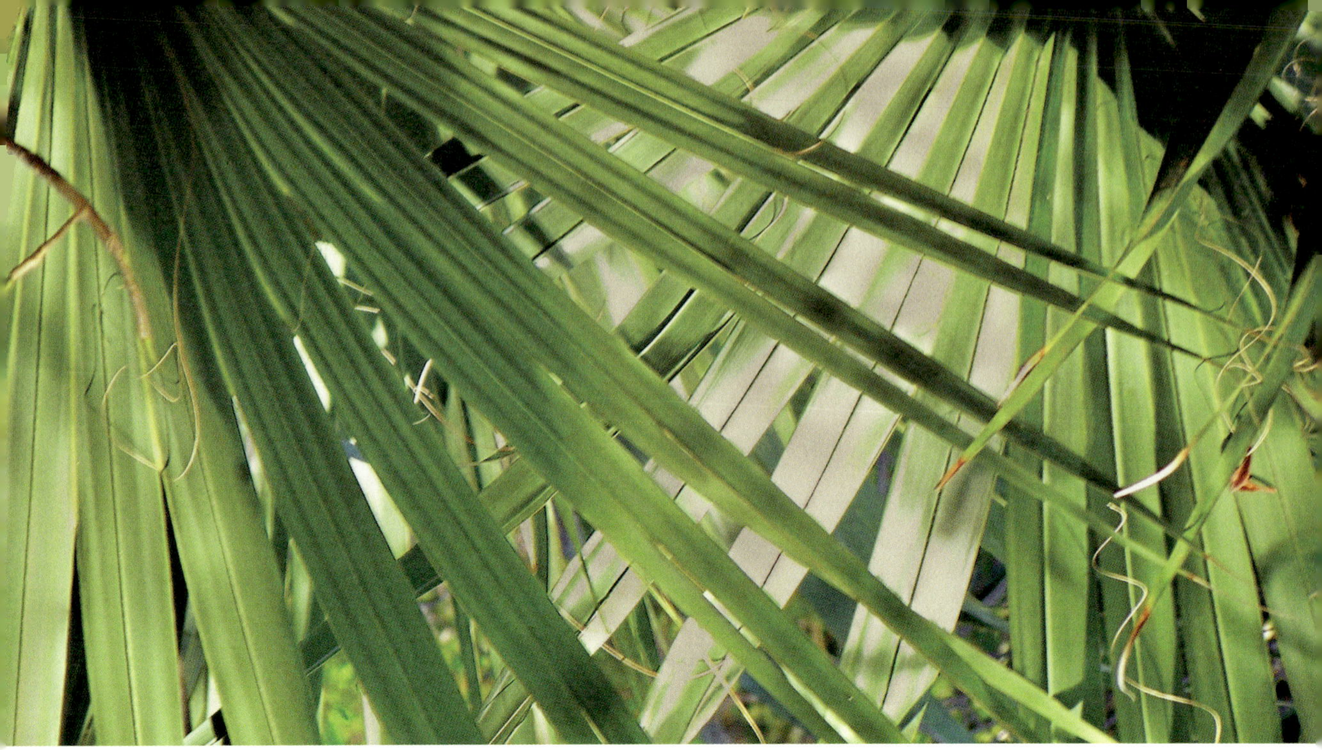

Saw palmetto is a supplement that comes from this plant. It has been proven to improve urinary tract health. Claims have been made that it can also prevent certain kinds of cancer, but no scientific research has proven this.

- A person substitutes supplements for prescription medicines. In most cases, supplements are not meant to treat illnesses. The word "supplement" means "add on to," not "cure"!
- A person takes too much of some supplements, such as vitamin A, vitamin D, and iron.

Special attention should also be paid to supplement use if you're going to have an operation. They can cause bad side effects before, during, and after surgery. For example, some may interfere with blood clotting and the effects of anesthesia.

NUTRITIONAL SUPPLEMENTS AND SPORTS

One of the most controversial uses of nutritional supplements is in sports. Instead of using supplements to provide missing nutrients, some athletes use them to get an advantage over other athletes. Sports are, by their

Make Connections: It's Not Just Guys

Most athletes who use nutritional supplements are male. Some female athletes also use these supplements to improve their strength and fitness, but for many girls and women, the hook is the chance to take a pill and lose inches and pounds. Advertisements are good at convincing people that there's some magic pill or substance that will change your body. But here are the best ways to get the body you want—if you want to be a stronger athlete, work hard and practice; and if you want to be a smaller person, work out more and eat less.

very nature, competitive, and some athletes are looking for a shortcut to stardom.

Doping is when athletes take drugs—such as steroids—to improve their performance. Another form of doping involves blood; by increasing their supply of red blood cells, athletes increase their energy and endurance levels. These are both illegal ways for an athlete to improve his performance; if he's caught, he could lose the chance to compete ever again—and he might even end up in prison.

Nutritional supplements aren't usually considered to be such a serious problem as doping. Some athletes use creatine and protein supplements to build muscle, both of which are legal. Creatine is popular with high school students who participate in football, gymnastics, hockey, and wrestling because it can increase muscle mass, help the muscles recover more quickly after exercise, and help athletes who need bursts of speed and energy. It's a protein that is naturally found in your body's muscle cells. When taken in larger doses than is found in the body, creatine can increase the rate of protein ***synthesis*** within your cells, giving you more energy and power. However, creatine does not have the same effect for everyone. Between 20 to 30 percent of athletes

Text-Dependent Questions

1. What are nutritional supplements?
2. How could you avoid the need for nutritional supplements?
3. What is one medical condition mentioned in this chapter that would require taking a nutritional supplement?
4. According to the sidebar, what are some reasons parents give their children nutritional supplements? Does scientific research support these reasons?
5. Describe some possible side effects of taking nutritional supplements.

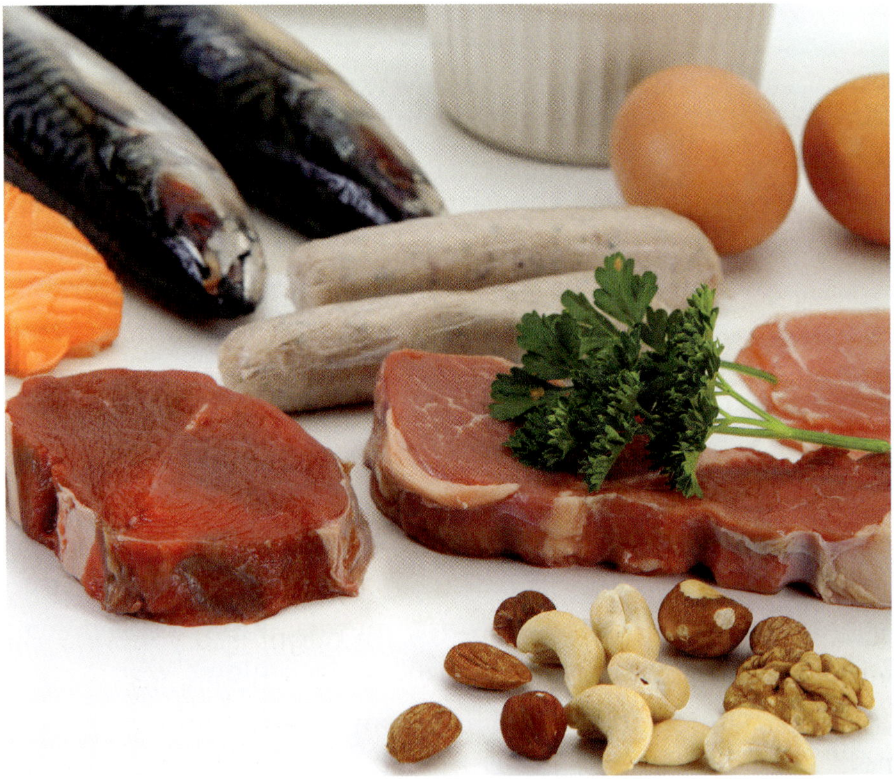

The best way to get the protein athletes need is by eating a healthy diet that includes foods like lean meat, fish, dairy foods, beans, and eggs.

Research Project

According to the chapter, young males often take nutritional supplements to have an edge against sports competitors, and young females do so to lose weight. Look at advertisements on line and in magazines. Make a list of products that claim to deliver one of these things. Then do some research, either online or in the library. Can these products actually deliver what they promise? Why or why not?

don't respond to creatine supplements. Because not enough research has been done into creatine's side effects, most doctors recommend that athletes who are seventeen or younger not take creatine. As for protein, your body needs it every day to be healthy. Eating protein immediately after a workout is a good idea, because it helps your muscles repair themselves after any damage. A protein shake can be a convenient way to get the protein that builds strong muscles. However, some doctors are concerned that young athletes could be consuming too many protein supplements. Protein shakes can contain a lot of sugar and other ingredients that could lead to weight gain.

If you're an athlete, the best use of supplements is to help fill any nutritional holes caused by a busy schedule of practice, games, and school. If you really don't have time to eat a healthy meal or snack before practice, for example, a protein shake might tide you over. Always check with your health-care professional before beginning to take nutritional supplements, though, and if you are already taking a nutritional supplement, be sure to let all your health-care providers—including your pharmacist—know. That way you can avoid any harmful interactions.

In the long run, though, here's the best route to take to reach your fitness goals—make a food and fitness plan, and then stick to it!

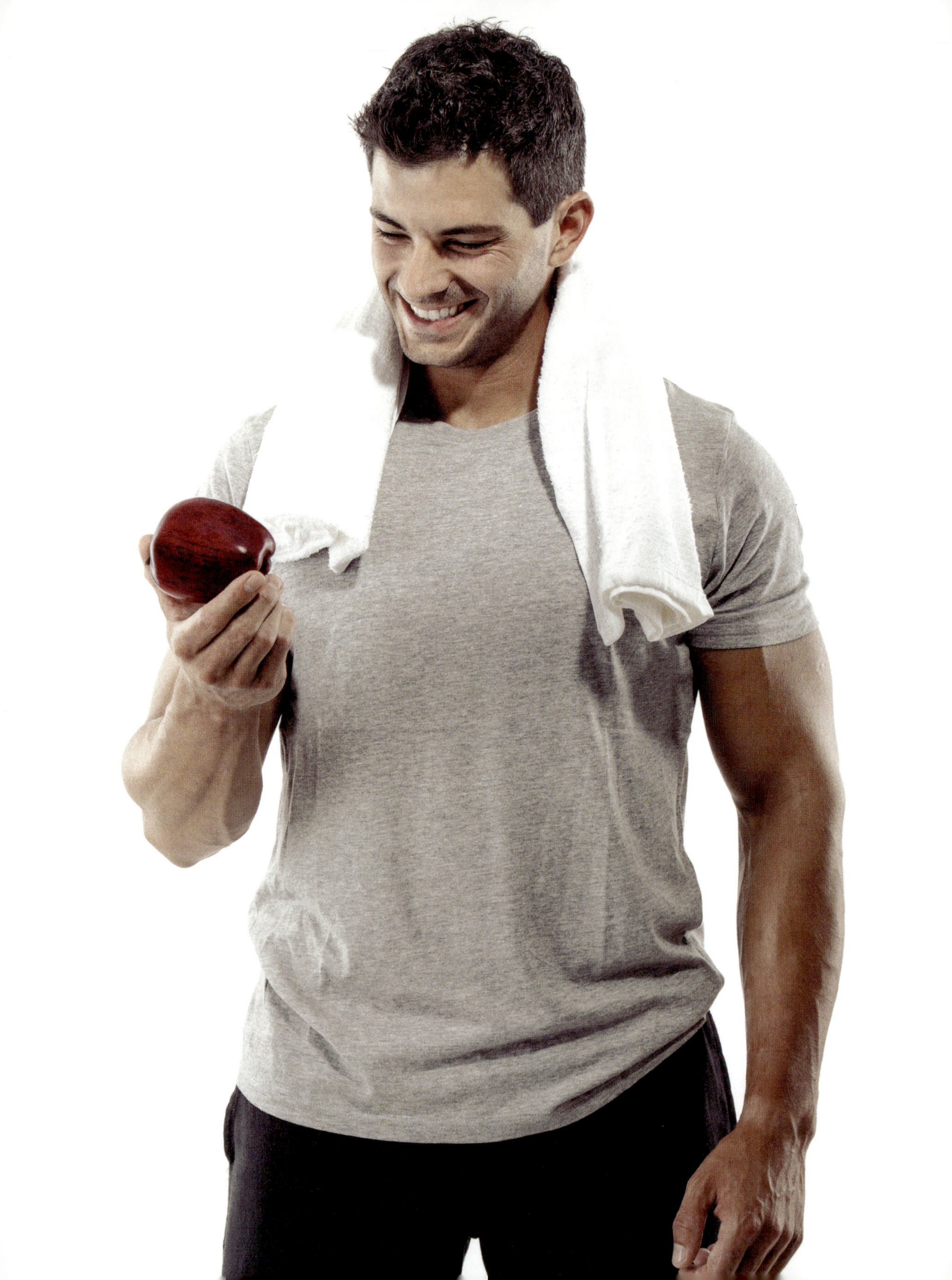

Chapter Four

Making a Food and Fitness Plan

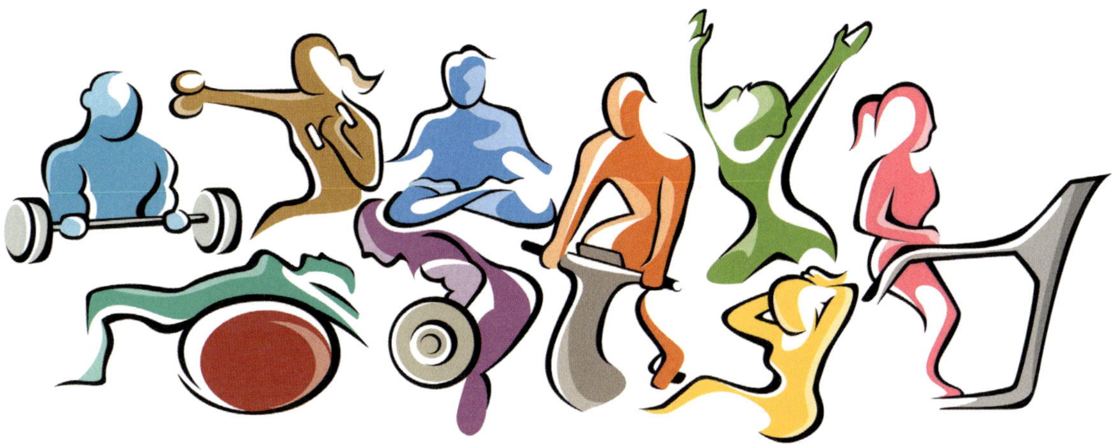

Part of being healthy and fit means being knowledgeable about your food choices. It's easy to just give up, of course, especially if you feel as though you have little control over the food choices at home and school. But there's a lot you can do, even if you're not the one who makes the menus!

Big projects are more easily accomplished when there is a plan in place. Planning ahead can help you anticipate problems and work out possible solutions before they occur. Planning can also make things easier to visualize. Just like other projects, using your knowledge about food to become fitter can be easier if you make a plan.

MYPLATE

A healthy diet must be balanced. A balanced diet is one that includes foods from all five food groups. Someone who eats a balanced diet is likely to have all the vitamins and minerals she needs to get through the day with energy to spare.

We used to hear a lot about the food pyramid, but in 2013, the USDA came out with a new picture to show how much of each food group people should eat every day. The picture shows a plate divided into four sections, each a different color. To the side of the plate is a blue glass.

Each section represents a food group. The green section on the left is labeled "Vegetables." It takes up a little more than one-fourth of the plate. The remainder of that side is labeled "Fruits." The right side of the plate is divided equally between a purple "Protein" section and an orange one marked "Grains." The glass is labeled "Dairy."

The purpose of dividing the plate into sections is to give you a visual reference of how much of each food group you should eat at each meal. It's the same information given in the text, but seeing a picture of it can make it easier to understand. Most of your plate should contain vegetables. There should be a little less of the other groups; fruit should take up the least amount of your plate. Over the day, half the grains eaten should be whole grains. And don't forget the glass represents all dairy, not just milk. Each section can have more than one food. For example, maybe you're having peas and carrots at a meal. They can share the vegetable space.

Your meal may not look like MyPlate all the time. In fact, it would be unusual if it did. Use MyPlate as a guideline for what you should eat over an entire day. Each day you should eat foods from all the groups.

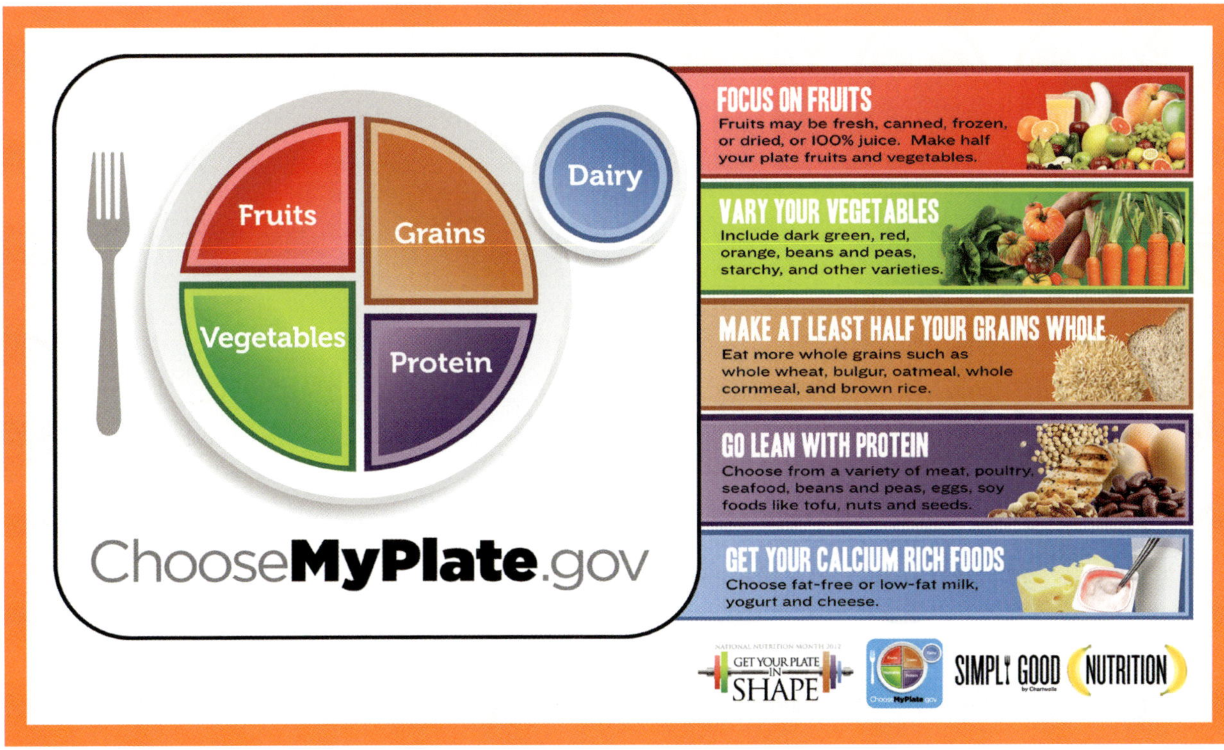

The USDA created MyPlate to help people understand how to choose a healthy diet.

If you don't have grains for a meal, make sure to make up for it at another meal or in a snack.

As discussed earlier in the book, some people have allergies or religious or philosophical reasons for not eating certain foods, such as meat. But remember, there are other protein sources you can choose from. And if you're allergic to dairy, add some kale or other calcium-rich vegetable to your food plan for the day. Using MyPlate to help plan meals will help you remember to keep your diet balanced. And keeping your diet balanced helps you be fit.

5 A DAY

Another popular nutrition program is called "5 a Day." Most experts say you should have five servings of fruits and vegetables a day. You may wonder how you could possibly fit in that many fruits and

Make Connections: SuperTracker

You can find several tools online to help you create a meal plan specifically for you and your needs. One of these is *SuperTracker* (www.supertracker.usda.gov/default.aspx). After you provide some information—including age, goals, and gender—a you-specific plan will be created. If you would rather not give out that information, you can use a general plan.

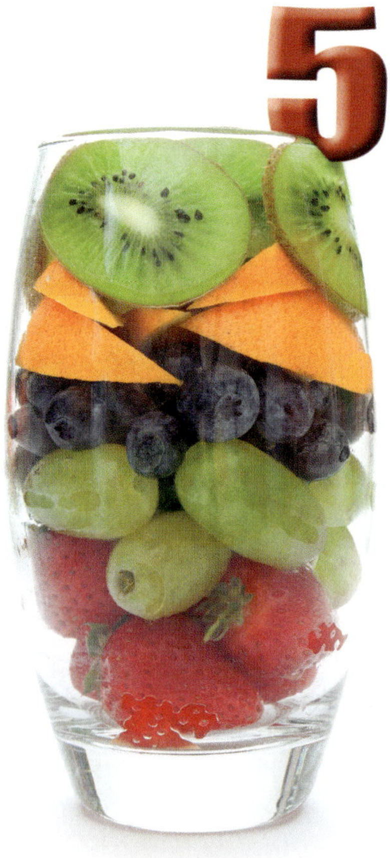

"Strive for Five," is another easy way to remember to try to eat five servings of fruits and vegetables each day.

Make Connections: The Latest in a Long Line

The USDA has set out dietary guidelines since 1894, when Dr. Wilbur Olin published them as part of a farmers' bulletin. Among other forms, the guidelines have appeared as the Basic 7 (1943–1956), the Basic Four (1956–1992), the Food Guide Pyramid (1992–2005), and MyPyramid (2005–2013). MyPlate is the latest version.

vegetables—but when you think of it in terms of your MyPlate, it seems more doable. The big question is, how much is a serving? Here are some guidelines.

- **Vegetables**: 1 cup of raw leafy vegetables; 1/2 cup of other vegetables, raw or cooked; 1/2 cup juice
- **Fruits**: 1 medium fruit (medium is defined as the size of a baseball); 1/2 cup chopped, cooked, or canned fruit; 1/2 cup small fruit, like berries or grapes; 1/2 cup juice
- **Meat, Poultry, Fish, Eggs**: 2–3 ounces of cooked lean meat, poultry, or fish (about the size of a deck of cards); 1 egg, 2 egg whites, or 1/4 cup liquid egg substitute
- **Beans and Nuts**: 1/2 cup cooked beans, lentils, or peas; 1/4 cup nuts; 2 tablespoons nut butter
- **Grains**: 1 slice of bread; 1 ounce of ready-to-eat cereal; 1/2 cup of cooked cereal, rice, or pasta
- **Milk, Yogurt, and Cheese**: 1 cup of fat-free or low-fat milk or yogurt; 1.5 ounces fat-free or low-fat cheese; 1/2 cup fat-free or low-fat cottage cheese

How many fruits and vegetables you should eat each day depends in part on gender and age. Here are guidelines for vegetables from MyPlate:

- toddlers 2–3: 1 cup
- children 4–8: 1 1/2 cups
- girls 9–13: 2 cups
- boys 9–13: 2 1/2 cups
- girls 14–18: 2 1/2 cups
- boys 14–18: 3 cups
- women 19–50: 2 1/2 cups
- men 19–50: 3 cups
- women over 50: 2 cups
- men over 50: 2 1/2 cups

MyPlate guidelines for daily fruit intake are

- children 2–3: 1 cup
- children 4–8: 1–1 1/2 cups
- girls 9–13: 1 1/2 cups
- girls 14–18: 1 1/2 cups
- boys 9–13: 1 1/2 cups
- boys 14–18: 2 cups
- women 19–30: 2 cups
- women 31–50: 1 1/2 cups
- women 51+: 1 1/2 cups
- men 19–30: 2 cups
- men 31–50: 2 cups
- men 50+: 2 cups

These amounts are for people who get at least 30 minutes of activity a day in addition to performing the activities of ordinary, everyday tasks. If you are more active, you can eat more.

Getting those 5 a Day into your food plan may be easier than you think. Have your first with your first meal of the day. Start the day with at least one serving of fruit. Make sure you also have vegetables at lunch and dinner. You know sometime during the day you'll want a snack. Make the most of your snack. It's a great way to get in another serving of fruits and vegetables. It will also give you a boost of energy when you may need it most.

When you think of fruits and vegetables, you may think of them as standalones—you eat them on their own or sometimes mixed together with other fruits or vegetables. But they can be so much more. Use them as ingredients in other things you like. Do you like soup? Combine vegetables you like with those you don't like so much. You'll notice your favorite ones more than those you are not so fond of. Grind up some slightly cooked vegetables, add an egg and some bread crumbs, broil or grill it—and you have a veggie burger.

We all can fall into a food rut, eating the same things over and over again. Promise yourself you will try something new every week. Is there a fruit or vegetable you have seen at the grocery store but never eaten? Ask whoever does the grocery shopping in your house if you could try it. Have you wanted to try a favorite fruit or vegetable in a different way? Here's your chance!

DEVELOPING A FITNESS PLAN

Educated food choices play an important role in being healthy and fit. But it takes more than eating a healthy diet. You need to get up and move.

In chapter 1, we took a look at the components of being fit—cardiorespiratory endurance, muscular strength, muscular endurance, body composition, and flexibility. Activities to develop these components should be included in your fitness plan. They should include a variety of exercises.

If you can join a gym, fine! But it isn't necessary. If you enjoy team sports, that's a great way to exercise. But again, you do not have to be part of a team. You just have to get up and move.

If you're like many people, you'll start out just fine. But then life happens, and you get busy. Before long, exercising becomes an

Text-Dependent Questions

1. Explain how can you have a balanced diet.
2. Describe how MyPlate is divided.
3. What is the 5 a Day program?
4. According to the chapter, what types of activities should be included in a fitness plan?
5. How much exercise do you need?

afterthought. So how can you stop this from happening? Here are some ideas.

Set Up a Schedule

You need to go to school or work at a certain time. You may not always like going, but you know it's something you have to do. So you get in the habit of going. You don't have to make a decision every day about whether to do it; you just do it. Do the same things with exercising. Make it a habit.

Get a Workout Buddy

You don't need a workout buddy—exercise can be something you do by yourself—but it can be fun to have someone to work out with. Plus, the other person can help keep you on track for your fitness goals.

Find Something You Like to Do

It's almost always easier to do things we like than things we don't. The same goes for physical activities. If you hate sports, then joining a team

Research Project

Using information in this chapter and what you find online and in the library, develop a food and fitness plan for yourself.

probably won't be the best choice for you. But what do you enjoy? If you like nature, maybe long walks outdoors would be a good form of exercise for you. Or if you hate getting up early, then maybe it's not such a good idea to try to set your alarm for 5 a.m. to go jogging. Instead, right after school might be a better exercise time for you. Find some activity you genuinely enjoy doing—and then find a time to do it that will work best with your schedule. When we do things we like to do, we're more likely to keep doing them.

HOW MUCH EXERCISE DO YOU NEED?

On average, children and teens between the ages of six and seventeen should exercise at least 60 minutes three times a week. Adults between eighteen and sixty-four should get in at least two and a half hours of exercise a week. Some experts say exercise can be done in several short sessions, while others claim it's necessary to work out at least 30 minutes at a time. Do what works for you.

Don't forget that you can add activity to your life in ordinary ways. Walk more, and use the stairs instead of an elevator. Just move.

It's worth it, in the long run. Your food and activity choices both play key roles in fitness—and being fit can mean a long, active life.

It's all up to you. The decision is yours!

FIND OUT MORE

In Books

Bijlefeld, Marjolijn, and Sharon K. Zoumbaris. *Food and You: A Guide to Healthy Habits for Teens.* Westport, CT: Greenwood, 2001.

Klimecki, Zachary, and Karen Bellenir (eds.). *Diet Information for Teens: Health Tips about Nutrition Fundamentals and Eating Plans.* Independence, KY: Omnigraphics, 2011.

Roizen, Michael F., and Mehmet Oz. *You: The Owner's Manual for Teens—A Guide to a Healthy Body and Happy Life.* New York: Scribner, 2011.

Salmon, Margaret Belais. *Food Facts for Teenagers: A Guide to Good Nutrition for Teens and Preteens.* Springfield, IL: Charles C Thomas, 2002.

Shanley, Ellen, and Colleen Thompson. *Fueling the Teen Machine.* Boulder, CO: Bull Publishing Company, 2010.

Online

Eating Well and Feeling Good
www.cyh.com/healthtopics/healthtopicdetails.aspx?p=243&id=2162&np=292

Food & Fitness
www.kidshealth.org/teen/food_fitness

Organic and Other Environmentally Friendly Foods
www.teenshealth.org/teen/food_fitness/nutrition/organics.html

Vegetarianism in Teens
www.pamf.org/teen/health/nutrition/veggieteens.html

Vitamins and Minerals
www.kidshealth.org/teen/food_fitness/nutrition/vitamins_minerals.html

SERIES GLOSSARY OF KEY TERMS

abs: Short for abdominals. The muscles in the middle of your body, located over your stomach and intestines.

aerobic: A process by which energy is steadily released using oxygen. Aerobic exercise focuses on breathing and exercising for a long time.

anaerobic: When lots of energy is quickly released, without using oxygen. You can't do anaerobic exercises for a very long time.

balance: Your ability to stay steady and upright.

basal metabolic rate: How many calories your body burns naturally just by breathing and carrying out other body processes.

bodybuilding: Exercising specifically to get bigger, stronger muscles.

calories: The units of energy that your body uses. You get calories from food and you use them up when you exercise.

carbohydrates: The foods that your body gets most of its energy from. Common foods high in carbohydrates include sugars and grains.

cardiovascular system: Your heart and blood vessels.

circuit training: Rapidly switching from one exercise to another in a cycle. Circuit training helps build endurance in many different muscle groups.

circulatory system: The system of blood vessels in your body, which brings oxygen and nutrients to your cells and carries waste products away.

cool down: A gentle exercise that helps your body start to relax after a workout.

core: The muscles of your torso, including your abs and back muscles.

cross training: When an athlete trains for a sport she normally doesn't play, to exercise any muscle groups she might be weak in.

dehydration: When you don't have enough water in your body. When you exercise, you lose water by sweating, and it's important to replace it.

deltoids: The thick muscles covering your shoulder joint.
energy: The power your body needs to do things like move around and keep you alive.
endurance: The ability to keep going for a long time.
flexibility: How far you can bend, or how far your muscles can stretch.
glutes: Short for gluteals, the muscles in your buttocks.
hydration: Taking in more water to keep from getting dehydrated.
isometric: An exercise that you do without moving, by holding one position.
isotonic: An exercise you do by moving your muscles.
lactic acid: A chemical that builds up in your muscles after you exercise. It causes a burning feeling during anaerobic exercises.
lats: Short for latissimus dorsi, the large muscles along your back.
metabolism: How fast you digest food and burn energy.
muscle: The parts of your body that contract and expand to allow you to move.
nervous system: Made up of your brain, spinal cord, and nerves, which carry messages between your brain, spinal cord, and the rest of your body.
nutrition: The chemical parts of the food you eat that your body needs to survive and use energy.
obliques: The muscles to either side of your stomach, under your ribcage.
pecs: Short for pectorals, the muscles on your chest.
quads: Short for quadriceps, the large muscle on the front of your upper leg and thigh.
reps: How many times you repeat an anaerobic exercise in a row.
strength: The power of your muscles.
stretching: Pulling on your muscles to make them longer. Stretching before you exercise can keep you flexible and prevent injuries.
warm up: A light exercise you do before a workout to get your body ready for harder exercise.
weight training: Exercises that involve lifting heavy weights to increase your strength and endurance.

INDEX

ABOUT THE AUTHOR AND THE CONSULTANT

Z.B. Hill is an author and publicist living in Binghamton, NY. He has written books on a variety of topics including mental health, music, and fitness.

Diane H. Hart, Nationally Certified Fitness Professional and Health Specialist, has designed and implemented fitness and wellness programs for more than twenty years. She is a master member of the International Association of Fitness Professionals, and a health specialist for Blue Shield of Northeastern New York, HealthNow, and Palladian Health. In 2010, Diane was elected president of the National Association for Health and Fitness (NAHF), a nonprofit organization that exists to improve the quality of life for individuals in the United States through the promotion of physical fitness, sports, and healthy lifestyles. NAHF accomplishes this work by fostering and supporting state governors and state councils and coalitions that promote and encourage regular physical activity. NAHF is also the national sponsor of Employee Health and Fitness Month, the largest global workplace health and fitness event each May. American College of Sports Medicine (ACSM) has been a strategic partner with NAHF since 2009.

PICTURE CREDITS

Fotolia.com:

8: Kenneth Man
11: CLIPAREA.com
12: nerthuz
16: high_resolution
18: andriigorulko
20: seralex
22: marilyn barbone
27: Monkey Business
30: Eva Gruendemann
32: crlocklear
36: Lilyana Vynogradova
38: Gennadiy Poznyakov
41: Es75
42: shimyra
44: Michael Roush
48: iko
52: Pixelbliss

1: Rongenel Robles | Dreamstime.com
25: Jkwchui
46: Bill Emrich | Dreamstime.com
51: www.choosemyplate.gov